Picking a Pedigree?

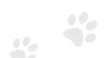

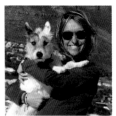

Michaela Strachan, TV wildlife presenter
I have been so shocked at what I've learned from Emma and her book. We have turned many pedigrees into freak shows, unable to breathe, give birth, walk properly or even fit their brains into their heads! It's hideous and it has to stop. Our pets should be companions not accessories designed to look cute, pretty, fluffy, fragile, funny. It's a world gone mad. If you love animals and care about their welfare, I urge you to read Emma's book before you get a pet so you can be sure you're not adding to the cruelty of in-breeding a designer animal. My advice, go for an adopted mongrel, as I call them, pavement specials! I did and she's the most amazing companion.

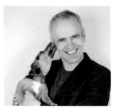

Dr Pete Wedderburn, *Daily Telegraph* vet
Emma has written the definitive guide to choosing a healthy puppy or kitten. She explains the evidence behind their health problems in a clear way that will be easily understood by new buyers and then outlines the easiest way to find a pet that will likely go on to become a healthy, long-lived adult. If you are considering getting a new puppy or kitten, make sure you read this book first.

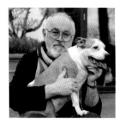

Peter Egan, actor and animal welfarist
I have become a bit of a 'purist' when it comes to the animals in my life. I've been rescuing dogs for over 20 years. All of them were discarded for one reason or another because of the careless attitude of those in our society who regard dogs or cats as property. The idea of ownership is a difficult one for me, it gives to the person, who owns the animal, rights which I do not agree with. They have the right to discard their animal if they don't want it anymore, or if it no longer suits their lifestyle. It's why I resist the term pet. My commitment to all animals in my life is complete. They are members of my family. I wouldn't refer to my child as a pet nor do I refer to my animals as such.

So when it comes to choosing a dog or cat, pedigree, for me, is not a priority. If, however, it were, I couldn't recommend Emma Milne's book more highly. If you are going to choose a pedigree know as much about the problems of making this choice as you can, it's all here in this book and will inform your choice. I think it's also good to know yourself; why are you choosing a certain pedigree, what are you asking of this animal in relation to your lifestyle? One thing which always amazes me is just how much animals have enriched my life. Their power to give is boundless and their power to forgive inspiring. They deserve the best from us. Give it to them by knowing them better

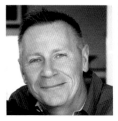

Lord Black of Brentwood, Patron, International Cat Care
Having a cat or a dog as part of your life is such a special, life-enhancing joy. They bring with them huge happiness, inspire unqualified love and deliver intense companionship. They enrich our lives in the way nothing else can. We owe them just one thing in return; to ensure we care for them, look after their needs and make sure they live long and happy lives. And that means not owning a pet that has been born to suffer, and which is simply a fashion accessory. There can be no excuse for choosing such an animal and perpetuating this trade in cruelty. Emma's comprehensive guide tells you everything you need to know about owning a pet which will be happy and healthy, and give you so much love in return. It is a must read – especially if you have ever been tempted by a designer cat or dog.

Picking a Pedigree?

How to Choose a Healthy Puppy or Kitten

Emma Milne BVSc MRCVS

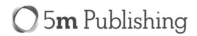

5m Publishing

First published 2018

Published by
5M Publishing Ltd,
Benchmark House,
8 Smithy Wood Drive,
Sheffield, S35 1QN, UK
Tel: +44 (0) 1234 81 81 80
www.5mpublishing.com

A Catalogue record for this book is available from the British Library

ISBN 9781912178896

Book layout by Servis Filmsetting Ltd, Stockport, Cheshire
Printed by Replika Press Pvt. Ltd, India
Chapter opening photos from Adobe Stock: Ch. 2 © Africa Studio;
Ch. 3 © adogslifephoto; Ch. 4 © dvr; Ch. 5 and 8 © Eric Isselée; Ch. 6 © Jne Valokuvaus;
Ch. 7 © Marc Dietrich; Ch. 9 © Erik Lam; Ch. 10 © Mopic; Ch. 11 © petrdlouhy; Ch. 12 ©
Michael Pettigrew; Ch. 13 © Andrey Kuzmin; Ch. 14 © verinize; Ch. 15 © fotorince.
Other photos by Emma Milne unless otherwise indicated

In memory of Pan and Badger.
The best friends a woman could ever wish for.

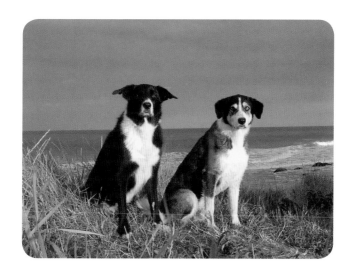

Contents

Foreword

I qualified from vet school in 1996. I had wanted to be a vet since I was about six or seven years old and, not being the sharpest tool in the woodshed, had worked extremely hard to get there. On one glorious sunny day in Bristol, bursting with pride, I swore an oath to '... pursue the work of my profession with uprightness of conduct and that my *constant endeavour will be to ensure the welfare of animals committed to my care.'*

I very soon started to realise that this oath was becoming increasingly about fixing man-made problems in people's beloved cats and dogs and I started to get very depressed about it all.

In 2007 I'd had enough and wrote a book about the terrible problems with pedigree cat and dog health, hoping to make some changes. In 2008 I was heavily involved in the BBC programme *Pedigree Dogs Exposed*. This powerful and heart-breaking documentary rocked the dog-breeding world. The BBC dropped its coverage of Crufts, a huge review into dog health was started and vets like me all over the world sighed a huge sigh of relief. Because surely now everything would change for the better.

A decade on and very sadly I fear things may have actually got worse. Vets find it as difficult as their clients when a beloved pet turns out to be sickly disaster. Helping owners through death and disease is always difficult, but when they are problems caused by our aesthetic desires it becomes quite simply soul-destroying. We feel like we are picking up the pieces because we are always too late. Virtually no one asks vets for advice *before* they get a pet.

So, I'm endeavouring once again to change things and help you, before you buy a kitten or puppy, to do everything in your power to choose a healthy pet. You might not like some of the things I'm going to say because you might have your heart set on a certain breed, but at least promise me you'll listen and reflect on your choices before you make a decision. Let's try and make your next pet a healthy, happy, enduring friend for you and your family.

Chapter 1

Making Friends

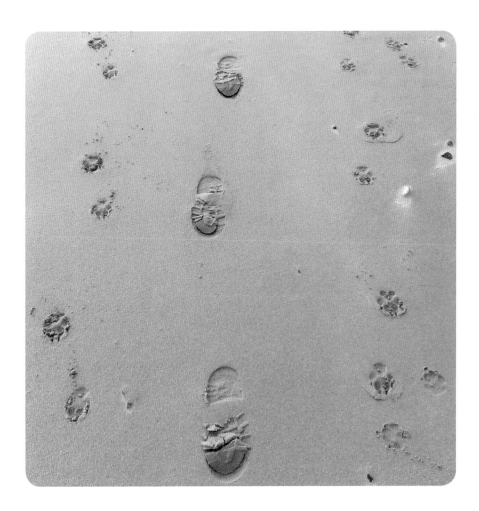

IN A CAVE IN FRANCE ARCHAEOLOGISTS HAVE FOUND THE FOOTPRINTS OF a child, estimated to be about eight years old, walking alongside the paw prints of a large dog-type animal. These footprints are thought to be about 26,000 years old. I love this fact. I absolutely adore dogs and the whole idea of how we started cohabiting makes me feel weirdly proud of both species. I'm all about teamwork and living in harmony on this beautiful planet of ours, so when species truly work together it's simply wonderful.

Lots of studies are still being done to try and figure out exactly how long man and dogs have been friends and exactly how domestic dogs developed from wolves or their common ancestors. It seems likely that as long as 40,000 years ago doggy-type animals started hanging around with us for mutual benefit. The animals got the benefit of the warmth from our fires and started to clear up the scraps that we didn't want. We started to get the benefit of extra eyes and ears on the lookout for predators and the natural pack-guarding instinct of those doggy ancestors. We gradually learned that if we hunted together we made a pretty good team and the friendship was sealed.

Cats evolved, probably, from a common ancestor of the African wild cat. Since then, well, they've used and abused us and from the earliest times they've tolerated us for our benefits! The more humans grew, cultivated and stored foods such as grain, the more we attracted one of the most successful families on the planet; rodents. Cats soon sussed out that hanging around the humans brought shelter in barns and an endless supply of tasty rats and mice. Humans, of course, got the mutual benefit of pest control in a very low maintenance way. As rodents have long been held as the devil incarnate when it comes to the spread of disease, cats were also pretty handy to have around.

We'll leave cats here for a while because until very recently cats and humans have simply grown together. They were ideal for what we needed, so we left them alone. They've crept closer over the years and wheedled their way into our homes and hearts, and on to our laps in some cases, but for thousands of years they stayed their same old moggie selves – cat-shaped, aloof, healthy and fit for the life that nature intended for them.

Dogs, on the other hand, had different qualities that man could exploit and this has turned out to be a foundation of some of the most fundamental and incredible changes in our modern-day pet dogs. Dogs were fast, fierce, intelligent, team players. As man developed we started to realise that some dogs by hazard were slightly better at one thing than another. It's not rocket science to see how we started to select dogs for different jobs.

If you breed two slightly larger dogs together you are likely to end up with bigger generations that may be stronger and more suitable for tackling large animals, such as deer and wild pigs. If you go in the other direction you can start to produce slightly smaller dogs that might fit down rabbit holes more easily.

If you pick the stronger, more aggressively loyal dogs you're likely to end up with dogs that have a stronger guarding instinct and are more frightening to your enemies. If you have an intelligent dog and breed it to a fast, fit dog you'll likely end up with dogs that are very good at herding and easily trained to round up animals you have no chance of catching or moving.

Guarding, herding and hunting; just three jobs for which we needed our dogs.

You can argue we needed slightly different types of hunting dogs depending on the prey; there are records of them being used for different jobs going back to ancient Egyptian times, around 2000 BC. So for argument's sake let's say that for around 36,000 years we were pretty happy with a handful of dog shapes and sizes. In the last century or so we have defined and named more than 200 totally distinct breeds of dog. To put that in perspective, if we've been friends with dogs for an hour, we've created virtually every recognised breed in the last *nine seconds.*

I think it's worth dwelling on this for a minute because once you start to really grasp what man has done to the domestic dog it starts to seem undeniably just a little bit wrong. If we managed for all those years happy to be friends with 'just dogs' what on earth happened in that final century?

What happened was we stopped needing them and we started just wanting them. Dogs are beautiful, wonderful animals to share your life with. Of course, over all those thousands of years man started to realise that dogs are actually lovely animals to have around. They make us feel safe and happy and loved. They don't judge us like humans do, they don't care what mood you're in when you get in from work, they don't care what your fashion sense is like or whether your ears stick out. They just love you and they keep on loving you until the day they die.

Humans, on the other hand, are a bit odd. We like to draw attention to ourselves, we are selfish, needy and stupid. We like to tinker with things and then show off about it and make other people think we are clever. So when we started having pet dogs, we started showing them to each other. And then we started deciding who had the best dog and we did this based on what they looked like, nothing else. We started saying that dogs that looked a certain way were better than other dogs. And so began our obsession with breed and looks, and without noticing it we took our eye off the ball that Mother Nature had juggled perfectly for millennia and we stopped judging them on how *healthy* they were. Soon all that mattered was the shape of their head, the exact length of their legs or whether they had the right spots in the right shapes and sizes to be considered 'desirable'.

The showing and breeding of dogs exploded at the end of the 1800s; the Victorians really went to town with it. They wanted special breeds of dog to distinguish their dogs from the lowly commoners' animals. Kennel Clubs started to spring up to organise dog registrations and run the shows and award the prizes. They set what's called the breed standards. This means they decide what a certain breed *should* look like and what constitutes the 'perfect' example of that breed in their view. It's a bit like a knitting pattern for dog breeders, except they're making arbitrary criteria for the body shape of a living, sentient mammal rather than a quirky item of fashion wear.

The American Kennel Club started in 1885 with just 19 recognised breeds. By the end of the 1800s there were already 55 and now it recognises well over 200. In fact, around 40 breeds were added from 2000–2016. Going back to our hour-long relationship with dogs, this equates to just over a second.

What people need to understand is that this is ridiculous and unsustainable. We have more than 200 physically different interpretations of the same species, and this is mind-boggling. Imagine if you did the same to any wild species. Imagine if we imposed the shape of a dachshund on a racehorse. Would we be outraged that it couldn't run or because we had abnormally affected its limbs with dwarfism? Or would we just think it was cute?

Every time you introduce another breed the others all have to become slightly more extreme versions of themselves. If you look back at pictures from the early dog shows, the ways the breeds have already changed is absolutely staggering. We need to remember this when we hear people say you can't change breeds. We already have, beyond recognition. And we need to be mindful of this when people say you can't get rid of a breed. We started with a handful, we didn't miss the breeds before we had them so we need to think very carefully about the ongoing health and welfare of the dogs and cats we've since created.

Now what I really would like people to start to do is think about nature's dogs and cats. Evolution is a *very, very* long process. The only times evolution cares what an animal looks like is if another animal of the same species finds it attractive enough to continue the genes, or if it's well enough hidden to avoid getting eaten. Evolution cares about who is best at finding food and water, finding a mate, living longest and producing the healthiest offspring that have the best chance of doing the same. It's called survival of the fittest for good reason. Breeds are a totally man-made concept and wouldn't exist in nature and, to be brutally honest with you, appallingly these days some breeds are literally just scraping an existence because of continued and almost constant veterinary intervention.

Recently I was researching wild types of relatives to dogs for a children's book. I wanted children to understand how dogs live in the wild to help explain their behavioural and social needs when they are kept as pets. Wild canids (the family to which the dog belongs) tend to have long muzzles, erect ears, bright, forward-pointing eyes, long legs and bushy tails. These include African wild dogs, wolves, coyotes, jackals, foxes and dingoes. Differences exist, but they all have these things in common and they are all highly successful species. *Not breeds, species.* I think we need to go back to thinking about our pet dogs as a species and ensure the species is healthy rather than getting hung up on breeds and looks.

So during the coming chapters, when you think about the generally accepted breeds of modern dog I want you to try and think back to natural canids and cats, evolution and survival of the fittest. By doing this you will tend to pick healthier body shapes and find beauty in the natural once again, rather than the sometimes unworkable but popular, man-made extremes.

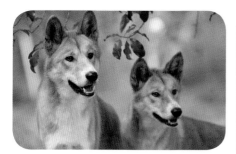

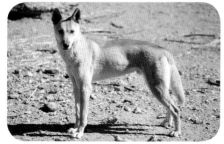

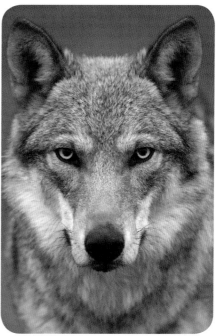

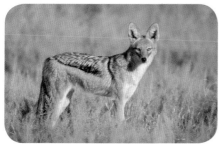

Figures 1.1, 1.2, 1.3, 1.4: Wild canids have erect ears, long legs and long muzzles. (photo: Adobe Stock)

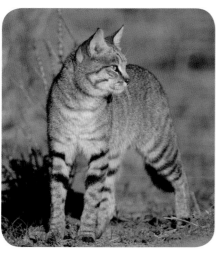

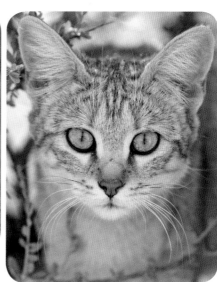

Figures 1.5, 1.6: And everyone knows what a cat should look like! (photo: Adobe Stock)

Chapter 2

Pedigree or Inbred?

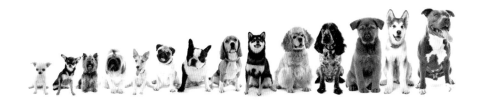

THE WORD PEDIGREE CONJURES UP ALL SORTS OF POSITIVE MENTAL images doesn't it? Royalty, the landed gentry, the best of the best. From beers to pet foods, the word is used to give brands some kind of distinction from the masses; connotations of being upper class somehow and better than all the rest. The *Oxford English Dictionary* defines the word 'pedigree' as:

1. The record of descent of an animal, showing it to be pure-bred.
   a. A pure-bred animal.
2. The recorded ancestry or lineage of a person or family.
   a. The history or provenance of a person or thing, especially as conferring distinction.

You'll notice that words such as 'pure' and 'distinction' are used. Being able to trace someone's lineage, or know that it has come from a distinguished background, is clearly seen as a good thing.

On the other hand, the word inbred conjures up all the opposite emotions. How many times have people sniggered about those who come from small, isolated areas and villages? The underlying theme to many of these jokes and snide remarks is that the inhabitants are inbred, having slept with close relatives too many times, producing offspring of little intelligence or with odd physical traits, such as a limp, a misshapen body or excessive hair.

Lots of vets have said to me that they would like to ask prospective owners if they would prefer a pedigree animal or an inbred one. Everyone's knee-jerk reply is, of course, that they would want a pedigree, not something that's inbred. The trouble is that they are absolutely the same!

As I said, pedigree cats and dogs are totally man-made concepts. Breeds have been created by breeding the same families and genetic lines together over and over again. For many years in the UK, and in many other countries, it has been widely accepted that it's fine to mate sisters and brothers, dads and daughters, mums and sons. In fact, there are some breeders who see this as the best way to ensure the 'purity' of their lines. This is inbreeding without a shadow of a doubt. At the surgery I have often been presented with a family's beautiful new puppy and with a flourish the owner produces the pedigree certificate, sometimes proudly telling me that they have paid extra for an even longer certificate. It's not until you glance down the family tree that you realise the same names are on it in many of the generations. It's difficult to share the joyous expectation the owner has that this is somehow proof of great things to come.

In most parts of the human population, inbreeding is frowned upon. It's caused historical blips in the past with problems such as the haemophilia in certain lines of the royal family of old. Inbreeding and the problems it brings with it are difficult to understand. Genetics is a bit of a minefield to navigate and get to grips with.

Evolution has, almost as if by accident, selected the best genes, whether that's the fastest, strongest, most camouflaged, most intelligent, it doesn't matter; as we said in the last chapter, nature selects animals and their genes based simply on who survives well enough to mate and produce offspring. The young of the best adapted carry the 'best' genes and are likely to go on to produce healthy young themselves.

Then you get to the dominant and recessive genes. Dominant genes are things including brown eyes in humans. A baby will get one gene (for simplicity's sake) for eye colour from each parent. If one is blue and one is brown the baby will have brown eyes because brown is dominant. Only when a baby gets two blues does it end up with blue eyes.

Some recessive genes are linked to diseases, but they generally don't get noticed because in nature these genes don't often end up together. The gene pool is an enormous ocean of variety, so the chances of two bad genes ending up in a mating and a baby are really small. When it does happen the young rarely survive long enough to reproduce, so the genes disappear even more from the population. It's genius!

However, when families, all carrying similar genes, get mated together time and again the ocean of variety starts to evaporate until you are left with a highly concentrated, stagnant puddle where the chance of recessive genes going forward is much higher. In pedigree, or should we say inbred, dogs and cats this is one of the reasons why there are some diseases that are very common in certain breeds and not others.

You can imagine disease-related genes as being a handful of Velcro-covered ping-pong balls floating in a giant lake full of millions of shiny, smooth ping-pong balls. The lake is the genetic diversity that normal populations have. The chances of the 'bad', sticky balls hitting each other and sticking together is pretty slim. When you take away the diversity by breeding related animals together it's like putting that same handful of bad ping pong balls in just a little bowl full of shiny ones. You'll soon end up with a big old clump of balls!

Now, and this is the crux, in fact you *can* have inbred animals that are *really* healthy. It all depends on *what you're selecting for*, and this is where we humans have totally taken our eye off the ball. Breeds of dogs and cats have been made by us and the most important criteria has always been *what the animals look like*. It is the appearance of the breeds that makes them immediately recognisable from the hundreds of others. The appearance is the defining characteristic of the breeds. Kennel Clubs and cat fancy associations have only come into being to manage the registration of purebred animals and it is those organisations that write the breed standards that breeders try to follow for the appearance of their dogs and cats.

I know nowadays there are plenty of breeders concerned with the declining health of pedigrees, and we will definitely go into that later, but for now we need to see what's happened to pedigree animals from the simplest starting point. In dogs and cats that is the fact that they have been bred with only their looks in mind.

So what about these healthy inbreds I mentioned? If you take animals that are incredibly healthy or resistant to disease and breed them together you are likely to end up with very healthy offspring. Dare I mention laboratory animals, but some lines of lab animals have been specifically bred to be the healthiest they can be. This type of breeding takes absolutely no notice of what the animals look like, it only selects for health.

What else has man selected for? Meat and milk. Again, a hot potato of a subject with all the welfare issues around intensive farming, but we have produced breeds of cattle that are milk factories. We only cared about udder size and milk production and we've ended up with astronomical milk volume. However, once again we didn't stop to think about what else we were selecting for, or the fact that a gigantic udder might not be very practical, or indeed comfortable, for the animal attached to it. The levels of foot disease and mastitis in dairy cows is a huge problem. We tinkered with nature, got greedy and got it wrong.

We made Belgian Blue cows. They are super muscly, which means huge amounts of meat, which makes lots of farmers and butchers and consumers very happy indeed. Oh but hang on, now the cows can't give birth because their babies' giant butts can't fit through their mums' little pelvises. We tinkered with nature, got greedy and got it wrong.

The fact remains we have manipulated nature for our gain whether it be for food or for rosettes, and we have to hold our hands up and admit we might just have messed it up. We know we can breed healthy animals, but we need to *stop caring what they look like.*

Not long after I qualified and had started making a little bit of a fuss about pedigree health problems I was invited to a meeting at the Kennel Club. We discussed health testing at length and I asked why hip scoring wasn't obligatory for breeds such as German shepherd dogs. We'll come back to the ins and outs of this test later, but for now a comment from that meeting has always stuck in my mind. The Kennel Club man told me that a certain kennel of police dogs in northern Europe had hip scored all their shepherds and selectively bred the condition out of their dogs. Surely getting rid of a crippling disease from a population of animals is something to be heralded, celebrated and shouted from the rooftops? In this instance, apparently, no. He looked at me with a serious and sad look on his face, shook his head forlornly and said, 'They didn't look like German shepherds anymore.'

I was so stunned by the ridiculousness of this, given as a reason not to get rid of disease, that for once in my life I was actually speechless. What *is* the answer to a statement like that?

By selecting for looks alone and inbreeding we have fundamentally gone against everything that Mother Nature and evolution have achieved in the last few million years. In that relative nanosecond of creating pedigree cat and dog breeds we have caused what I call the devolution of these species and we should be very ashamed of ourselves.

There are thousands of vets all over the world, myself included, who have dealt, time and again, with the heartbreak of families losing their animals. It's one of the hardest but most important parts of our job. When this happens after a long and wonderful life it is terribly sad, but it is part of the cycle of nature and, although it's unbearably hard, you can come to terms with it. What is impossible to come to terms with is when you have to euthanase a young animal or watch a family and their pet go through multiple surgeries to improve a poor quality of life simply because the animal is a certain breed. Have no doubt, as I said, breeds do not exist in nature and some of our current breeds are only scraping by because of veterinary intervention.

With this book I desperately want to help you make the right decisions when it comes to getting a puppy or kitten so I need you, in the coming chapters, to completely forget everything you think you know about breeds, forget which breed of dog or cat you were thinking of getting and open your mind to what I am about to say. By the end of the book I'd like you to have your eyes open to what different body shapes mean to the animals themselves, *not* what they mean to us. We've all played our part in getting to the current sad level of ill health in cats and dogs, but it is you, the future puppy and kitten buyers, that wield the most unbelievable power, way more than vets and breeders. You see, if you only choose the healthiest animals the demand for the debris of our tinkering will disappear and animal welfare will skyrocket overnight. I'm counting on you.

Chapter 3

Short Faces, Big Eyes and Curly Tails

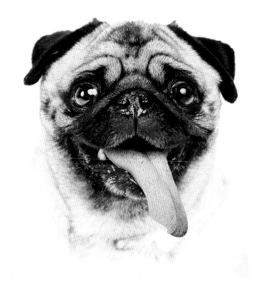

I WANT TO START WITH THIS BODY SHAPE FOR TWO REASONS; ONE IS THAT these animals are considered unbelievably cute and are hugely popular these days, and secondly this body shape causes possibly more suffering than any other and is the epitome of what we have done to cats and dogs. Remember to keep an open mind and forget what you think you know or want!

Short Faces

Before we embark on this chapter it's worth having a good look at Figure 3.1 and 3.2. It's easy to miss that there are two animals in each one. These photos, when you look closely, show a short-faced (brachycephalic, or brachy for short) animal superimposed on to a normal one. You will probably be shocked at

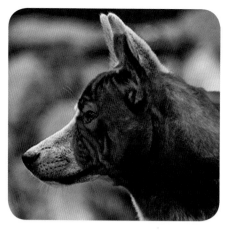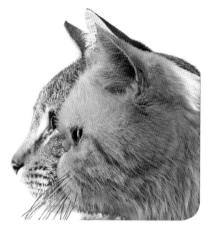

Figures 3.1, 3.2: (Photo: Cassie Smith; International Cat Care)

how much we have effectively amputated the faces of these animals by selective breeding.

The popularity of brachy breeds, especially dogs, has exploded in recent years with the French bulldog set to overtake the Labrador as the most popular breed in the UK. There are lots of brachy breeds, including boxers, bulldogs, pugs, Pekes, Japanese chins, mastiffs, Newfoundlands, Shar-Pei, Boston terrier, shih-tzus, King Charles spaniels, Chihuahuas, Persian cats, British and exotic shorthair cats, Scottish fold cats, and the list goes on.

As with many things in life, there is a spectrum when it comes to how short-faced animals are. Suffice to say that in general the shorter your face (if you're a dog, cat, or even rabbit for that matter), the more problems you are likely to have. The sad fact is that the most popular brachy breeds at the time of writing are some of the most extreme; English and French bulldogs and pugs.

There have been some fascinating studies into why people think flat-faced animals are so cute. When some animals such as mammals (including humans) are born they have a slightly flatter face than an adult, even in the long-nosed dog breeds, and they tend to have relatively large eyes for the size of their head. Because mammals are largely nurturing animals we have a strong drive to care for our young and nurture them. We find baby animals much more appealing in some ways than adults, which is one reason many animals are rehomed once they are no longer considered cute.

You can see then that the breeds that have been selected more and more to have shorter and shorter faces and larger and larger eyes have a look that some people find absolutely adorable. Better a baby face than a wolf in your living room, right?

Many of the flat-faced breeds were selected for slightly shorter faces right at the start of all this because of perceived benefits for their jobs. Supposedly having a slightly shorter face for a bulldog meant they could still breathe through their nose while hanging on to the side of a bull. Sadly, as you'll see, a great many of these animals can't breathe at all now, especially through their non-existent noses.

We are so used to the look of different breeds now that we never stop to think about the impact of what that body shape means. Lots of owners of short-faced dogs, for instance, accept that it's normal for their pet to snore when sleeping and make snorting noises when they are awake. In fact, some owners find it incredibly endearing. Normal dogs don't always snore and never snort or gasp unless they are ill; once you understand the reason the brachys do it tends to change your mind about how cute it is.

The first veterinary paper about the health problems in brachy dogs was written in 1934, around 60 years after the creation of the first Kennel Club and the development of breed standards. When you look at photographs of brachy dogs from back then they are virtually unrecognisable by today's extreme standards and their health has certainly declined even more.

To understand the implications completely we need to start at the nose and go all the way to the tip of the tail. Many of the problems in the head and neck contribute to something called BOAS. This stands for brachycephalic obstructive airway syndrome, which sounds very complicated, but is basically a collection of issues that tend to affect how well brachy animals can breathe or not as the case may be. As you'll see, the poor breathing is, of course, the most severe problem, but is just one thing among many from which these animals suffer.

If we start at the beginning, the first thing you encounter is the nose. Normal dogs and cats have wide open nostrils, while the brachys tend to have varying degrees of what's called stenotic nares. This simply means narrow nostrils. All of these changes are on a spectrum, but the more extreme ones have a nose that is virtually clamped shut compared to a normal animal.

Now this may not seem like a very big problem, but it affects dogs and cats more than you might think. We are all used to seeing dogs pant and breathe through their mouths, but you may be surprised to know that cats hate mouth-breathing and only do it if they are in respiratory distress, have a medical problem or are incredibly stressed or scared. Having nostrils that are so narrow for a cat that they have to mouth-breathe is far from natural or enjoyable for a cat (see Figures 3.3–3.6). Sadly, because cats are very good at just sitting still when they are compromised many of these issues can go unnoticed by their owners. Just because they can't climb the curtains doesn't mean they don't want to!

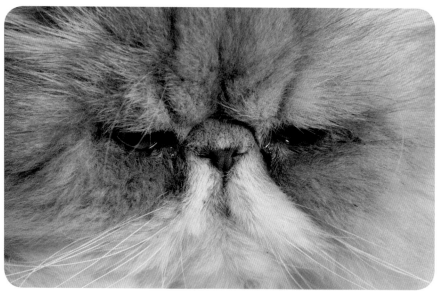

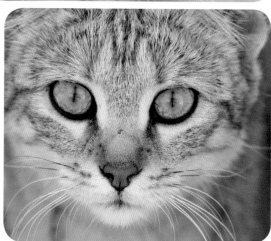

Figures 3.3, 3.4, 3.5, 3.6: Notice the tightly folded skin and how the whole position of a brachy cat's nose has totally changed compared to a normal cat. (Photo: Adobe Stock)

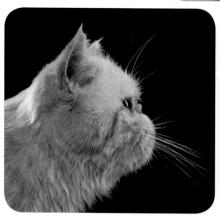

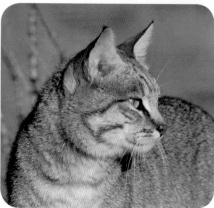

In dogs it might not seem too bad either because they really don't mind mouth breathing when they have to, such as when they need to increase their air intake when they exercise or actively use panting to cool down. The first thing to say about this is that we mouth breathe too when we exercise, but sometimes it's good to use a little empathy. It's not pleasant when you have a cold and your ability to nose-breathe is suddenly denied to you. When you are resting and sleeping it's definitely preferable to breathe through your nose, and the same is true for dogs (see Figures 3.7–3.10). It's actually quite difficult for a dog to sleep and breathe through its mouth, but we'll come to that later.

Research in recent years has actually uncovered a long-held misconception when it comes to dogs and their panting. For years we have believed that when dogs pant they breathe quickly in and out through their mouth, passing air over the large, blood-filled tongue, using this big surface area to cool down the blood

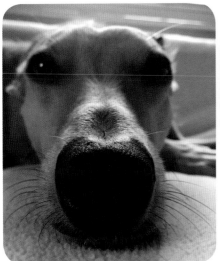

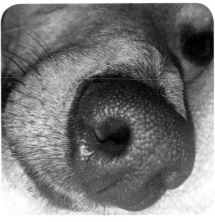

Figures 3.7, 3.8: A beautifully open normal nose compared with ... (Photo: Anna Porter)

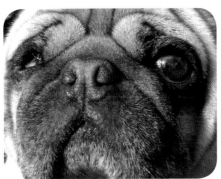

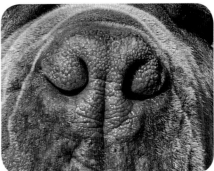

Figures 3.9, 3.10: ... a clamped shut brachy one. (Photo: Kate Price; Adobe Stock)

and therefore the dog. In fact, this is not true and the new findings show another critical reason why noses are so important to dogs.

When you go a bit beyond the nostrils you come to the middle third of the dog's nose and this turns out to be a truly wonderful thing. This area is absolutely packed full of little structures called conchae or turbinates. They have a huge surface area if you could lay them out flat, they are covered in beautiful, shiny mucosa and they are so incredibly evolved that although they are packed in and convoluted they never touch each other or rub together. The surfaces are constantly moistened with special fluid and the turbinates have a very high blood supply. We now know that when a dog pants virtually *none* of the air inhaled is through the mouth, it all goes into the nose. The cooler outside air passes over these wet, blood-rich surfaces and the dog is cooled down. The effect this area has on body temperature is enormous and, critically, keeps the brain cool. In Figure 3.11 and 3.12, the blue oval shows the combined area for cooling. As you can see, in brachy animals there simply isn't room for it. As a result of this some brachy dogs start panting at temperatures around 10 degrees Celsius lower than normal dogs. It's also the reason that many such animals are prone to heat exhaustion and collapse, because they simply can't stop their body temperature from becoming critically high.

It's not just the nose that has suffered when it comes to space requirements. A specialist in BOAS surgery has likened the brachy head to moving from a 200 sq m apartment to a 20 sq m apartment, but having to take all your furniture with you. You see, as we have selected for shorter and shorter jaws and faces the rest of the tissues and structures in there have stayed the same; teeth, tongue and soft palate.

Dental problems are huge in brachy animals. The jaws are so short in many cases that the teeth have to rotate or grow sideways to fit in the mouth. Most of the breeds are also 'supposed' to be undershot, which means that their bottom jaw is longer than the top, a totally unnatural phenomenon in cats and dogs. All of this means that the way teeth normally fit together doesn't happen. It becomes difficult for some dogs and cats to even pick food up, let alone chew it. Many animals have such bad alignment of their teeth that they have severe trauma to their mouths where teeth impinge on the other structures, including the lips and hard palate. A specialist friend of mine has seen cases so severe that the molars have ended up inside the dog's nasal cavity because there was nowhere else for them to go. The more mild cases are obviously less traumatic, but every single undershot or brachycephalic animal will have some degree of dental disease/malocclusion (see Figures 3.13–3.20). To quote veterinary dental specialist Dr Fraser Hale:

'It is absolutely fair to say that every brachy dog and cat has a malocclusion virtually by definition. The only truly normal occlusion is found in a mesocephalic head (medium-length head) – end of story.

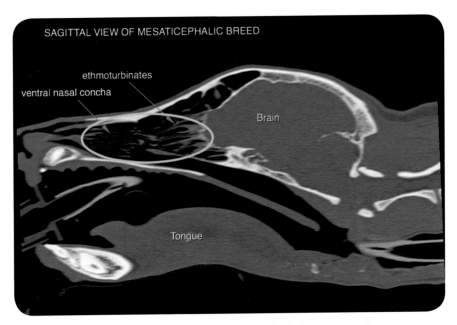

Figure 3.11: A normal dog with a huge area devoted to cooling conchae/turbinates.

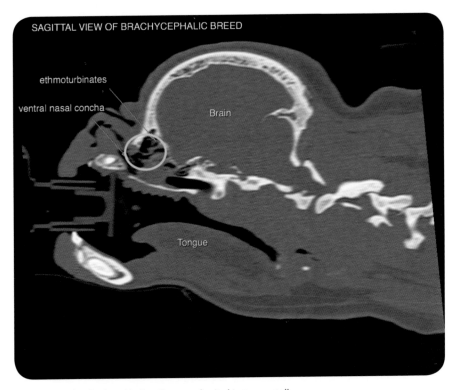

Figure 3.12: A brachy dog with virtually no conchae/turbinate area at all.

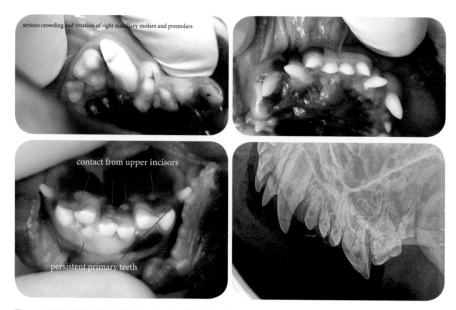

Figures 3.13, 3.14, 3.15, 3.16: Crowded teeth in a brachy mouth either struggle to erupt or have to rotate to fit in. (Photo: Dr Fraser Hale)

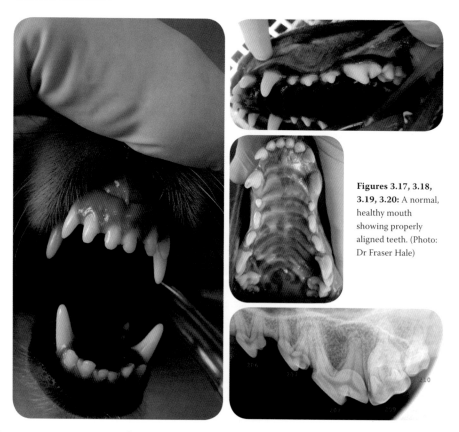

Figures 3.17, 3.18, 3.19, 3.20: A normal, healthy mouth showing properly aligned teeth. (Photo: Dr Fraser Hale)

In brachycephalic animals, the jaws are too short and in the vast majority of cases, the top jaw is dramatically shorter than the bottom jaw so nothing is where it should be. I occasionally see a brachycephalic dog or cat in which the relationship between the upper and lower jaws is fine because they are both too short to the same degree. This still results in crowding issues, dramatically increasing the risk for periodontal disease. My contention is that it is not possible to have a truly healthy mouth in a brachycephalic head unless the animal is congenitally missing most or all of its teeth.'

It's worth taking the time to reflect on this. *Every* brachy animal and every breed standard that asks for an animal to be undershot is potentially selecting *for* lifelong dental problems, pain, discomfort and abnormality.

You may have seen photographs of brachy dogs sitting or lying with their tongues poking out. These photos are shared endlessly on social media as cute and appealing. The fact is that in many of these dogs their tongues actually just don't fit in anymore. Remember all that furniture we mentioned you had to take when you downsized from your nice big apartment? Well the tongue is one giant settee. One of the flattest-faced dogs you'll find is the Japanese Chin. I was told by one breeder-turned-health campaigner that it is not unheard of for some breeders to request the tip of the tongue be removed surgically because it is seen as a fault in the show-ring if it protrudes!

As we go further back you come to the soft palate and things start to get even more dangerous. The soft palate is a clever little thing that helps do things such as closing off the nasal passages when you swallow food and helps protect the airway. This too is a piece of furniture that didn't shrink when the apartment got smaller.

In many brachy animals the soft palate is too long and gets sucked into the trachea (windpipe), causing a partial obstruction a bit like an over-long curtain that constantly gets stuck in the door when it opens. Obviously at exercise this is a huge issue as the whole airway becomes even more compromised.

Once you've clambered over the furniture you've piled into your new, tiny flat and hauled the curtain out of the door, let's say you decide to check outside that back door that leads to the alley that you want to use as a quick getaway in an emergency. This would be your brachy animal's larynx and trachea.

The larynx is the sturdy solid thing that is the start of your trachea and is where your 'voice box' lives. In dogs and cats there are two little saccules that sit near the entrance to the larynx. No one is very sure what they are for, but in brachy animals they tend to become everted or turned inside out. This might be due to the increased effort that is needed for breathing, placing more pressure on all the parts of the airway and eventually pulling these saccules out of their little pockets. Whatever the cause, if and when they do become everted they become another structure blocking air flow into the trachea. Shall we say the previous tenant left two armchairs blocking your back door?

You eventually climb over the armchairs into the emergency alley to find that it is barely big enough for a child to flee down, let alone a grown adult. The icing on the brachy cake is that for some reason we seem to have unwittingly selected for very narrow tracheas relative to the animal's size.

When you add all these things together you have an airway that is quite literally compromised and deficient at every single level. As I said earlier, it's quite difficult for dogs to sleep with their mouth open, but for some brachy animals it is a matter of life and death. As well as the 'cute' pictures of brachy dogs with their giant tongues poking out there is a very disturbing number of 'hilariously funny' videos circulating on social media of brachy dogs falling asleep sitting up and then falling over. Among these are videos of animals falling asleep leaning on things, or while playing with toys and bones. The comments and smiley face emoticons that accompany the endless shares is appalling once you understand why it is happening.

The fact is that with all the extra soft tissue and obstructions in their airways many of these animals find that as soon as they lie down and relax their airway is sealed shut. They can actually only breathe when they are alert and standing in a way that keeps their neck stretched out, mouth open and airway aligned. The unbelievably sad truth is that these animals fall asleep sitting up because they are exhausted from trying to stay upright. As for toys and bones, you'll see they are hollow toys, such as Kongs. These poor creatures have learnt that if they fall asleep with a hollow toy or bone wedged in their mouth they can still breathe and sleep. Please don't share these videos.

Of course, some animals have only one or two parts affected and there is, as I said, a huge variety in severity between, and within, breeds *but* you don't get BOAS in normal dogs and that is the most important statistic for me. For almost a century we have known that the brachy shape is detrimental to health and welfare and yet we have bred them to be more and more extreme, and their popularity is only growing.

A team at Cambridge University has started doing quite unique studies on brachy dogs by placing them in a large, clear chamber that measures air flow and breathing patterns without interfering with the animals at all. The researchers have been trying to get an idea of the level of the problems. Animals have an examination beforehand, have a short exercise period and are then measured and examined again using the chamber. BOAS is graded from 0, totally normal respiration, to III, severely affected or life-threatening problems. As you can see from Figure 3.21, the levels of disease in the three most popular breeds is horrifying. Pugs are worst affected, with only around 5% being grade 0, and almost a fifth of dogs are grade III. This

Cambridge Conformational Study: BOAS Grading

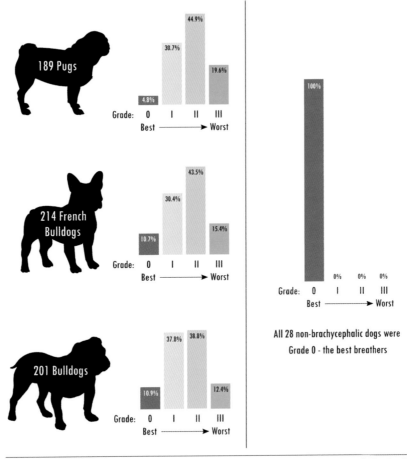

189 Pugs

4.8% 30.7% 44.9% 19.6%

Grade: 0 I II III
Best ——→ Worst

214 French Bulldogs

10.7% 30.4% 43.5% 15.4%

Grade: 0 I II III
Best ——→ Worst

201 Bulldogs

10.9% 37.8% 38.8% 12.4%

Grade: 0 I II III
Best ——→ Worst

100% 0% 0% 0%

Grade: 0 I II III
Best ——→ Worst

All 28 non-brachycephalic dogs were Grade 0 - the best breathers

Brachycephalic numbers from Table 2; *Conformational risk factors of brachycephalic obstructive airway sydrome (BOAS) in pugs, French bulldogs, and bulldogs*, Liu et al., 2017. Control numbers from Table 2; *Whole-body barometric plethysmography characterizes upper airway obstruction in 3 brachycephalic breeds of dogs*, Liu et al., 2016. BOAS grading - Grade 0: BOAS free; Grade I: mild BOAS with mild respiratory noise but no exercise intolerance; Grade II: moderate BOAS requiring weight control and/or surgery; Grade III: severe BOAS requiring immediate surgery.

Figure 3.21: BOAS scores for three popular breeds. (Graph: Cassie Smith)

is a travesty for health and welfare. You'll also note that every single non-brachy dog that was tested was a grade 0. The study is ongoing so the numbers tested will grow and the data may change. For now it seems clear the breeds are in trouble.

One very important thing to remember when it comes to BOAS is that it is a progressive disease. This means that it is rarely very obvious in young animals and becomes more and more severe with age. This is very important when you are looking for a good breeder if you do decide to go down this dangerous road. None of these dogs should be bred from before the age of about three years because you simply can't know before then if they are likely to go on to develop the disease.

We'll look at health testing in general and what else you can do to find the healthiest examples later.

A final point to make here is the added impact that being fat has on these animals. Being fat increases fatty soft tissue amounts in many places, including the neck. We've described in detail the constrictions in the airways of these animals, but if you have a fat brachy this is exacerbated even more. The extra tissue around the airways can compress them even more. It's imperative that brachy animals should be kept slim. You'll probably be as shocked as me to learn then that the UK breed standard for the pug, the worst brachycephalics of all, says that they are '... never to appear low on legs, nor lean nor leggy.' Never to be lean. This is totally unacceptable. To have a breed standard for any animal that calls for obesity is promoting cruelty; for this breed it's practically a death warrant. True to this, the photo in the 2017 KC updated breed standards book shows its ideal pug. It is unquestionably obese.

Sadly, studies have also shown that more than half of owners of these animals can't recognise signs of respiratory problems in their animals, probably because it is normalised so much. You hear of people saying they simply couldn't get to sleep without the comforting snore coming from their brachycephalic dog. One specialist I spoke to said that one thing they found so sad was the astonishment of owners after their animals had had surgery on their airways because they simply hadn't realised beforehand that they couldn't breathe.

For now we must move onwards and, as if the BOAS and dental problems weren't enough to be concerned about with these dogs and cats, we move next to look at the eyes, facial skin folds, intestinal problems and curly or stubby tails, too.

Big Eyes, Big Heads and Folded Skin

The problems with big eyes and folded skin go hand in hand in these animals. As we said with the tongue and soft palate, the skin on the head has not short-ened with the bones. This means that many of these dogs and cats have skin folds around their nose and bulging eyes that are prone to infections and sores. We'll be discussing skin folds and why they are a problem in more detail in Chapter 5, but I mention them here because they are a common feature in brachy animals and many owners go to extraordinary lengths to alleviate the problems associated with them. As we said with the accepted snoring, the skin care routine for many brachy owners is a completely normal, accepted part of the daily routine for these pets. How many normal dogs and cats require a daily face wash?

So what of those big eyes that we seem programmed to adore? The problem with animals with big eyes is that the eyes haven't actually got any bigger, they are just more prominent. It may be obvious to say, but let us not forget that eyes are pretty important to animals that live in any level of light. For predators such as dogs and cats they are absolutely essential for helping locate prey, judging distances and getting around in general. Evolution has made sure that natural eyes are, understandably, very well looked after.

Normal dog and cat eyes sit deep inside a rounded socket of bone, well protected from accidental injury. They have a constant supply of tears to keep them moist and help remove dust and dirt. When something does get in the eye, the tear production increases to help wash the dirt away. The eyelashes are a constant filter for larger debris, and the action of blinking cleans and protects the eyes as well. Tear fluid is effortlessly transported away into the nose by the nasolacrimal duct, a tiny tube that connects the eyelid to the nasal cavity. Eyes are a thing of wonder. A true triumph of nature. And then man came along!

The way we have made eyes in these animals look bigger is simply by exposing them. As we have selected for flatter and flatter skulls and faces we have made the eye sockets shallower and shallower. The eyes now bulge out, sometimes showing large areas of the white of the eye, mostly hidden in normal animals. Because the eyes bulge out, they are much more prone to disease and injury.

Many websites and breeder advice for these breeds caution against any pointy objects in the house in case the eyes get injured. I once spent a weekend at a pet show doing some promotion for my children's books, so I had been put on a stand in the kids' zone. At one point a bored little girl started having some great fun using the straw that had fallen from the straw-bale seating as confetti. She twirled around and watched, enchanted as it settled around her. This was brought to an abrupt end when a worried French bulldog owner asked her to stop in case her dog's eyes got injured. This is *not* normal.

Owing to the deranged shape of the face, the nasolacrimal duct in many of these animals is also now distorted. Its path is deviated, it can get crushed and kinked and prone to blockages. This means that many of these animals have tear staining on their faces because their tears simply overflow instead of draining away. Many people are led to believe it is normal. It is seen as normal for some breeds, but it is *not* normal for a healthy cat or dog. As nutritional advisors, we sometimes get phone calls from vets who have been told by clients they have heard that food can cause tear staining, or to ask if there is a food that can stop it. It's all nonsense. The breeds we are phoned up about that are brachycephalics and they have tear staining because their heads are deformed and their tears overflow.

Perhaps the most shocking thing about the big eyes is that sometimes they can come out. Unlikely as this may sound, there are many documented cases of brachy animals' eyes that have come out when they have been restrained for nail clipping, simple grooming or veterinary procedures, such as being held for anaesthetics. This

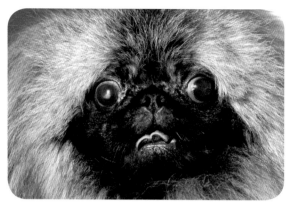

Figure 3.22: Exposed, bulging eyes are highly prone to injury. (Photo: David Gould)

is a minority, of course, but it is certainly not unheard of and something that we should find totally outrageous and stop selecting for immediately.

As the eyes bulge out in these dogs they are more prone to accidental injury (see Figure 3.22), but they also tend to be drier than normal eyes because the eyelid coverage is reduced. Dry eyes are uncomfortable and prone to ulcers that don't heal well. The skin folds around the face are often an inherent cause of damage and pain to the eyes (see Figure 3.23). In many of these animals you'll notice that the skin folds bulge up towards the exposed eyes. If any of you have ever had an eyelash in your eye you'll know how painful this is, so to have hairs impinging on your eyes constantly must be simply horrible.

Chronic ulceration and trauma is a major cause of eyes having to be surgically removed in these animals and seeing brachy animals with one eye is surprisingly common compared with normal animals (see Figure 3.24).

Another problem some of these breeds tend to have is a condition called cherry eye. Cats do get cherry eye, but it is much more common in dogs. Tears are produced by a number of different glands and one of these is in the third eyelid. This is an extra eyelid that you will see the rim of just across the inside corner of the eye. One of the tear glands sits inside this eyelid and sometimes it pops out and is seen as an obvious reddish-pink protrusion. It happens in some non-brachy breeds too, but is quite common in breeds such as bulldogs.

You will often see and hear owners and breeders of these dogs publicly berating some vets as money-grabbers and practically as monsters when it comes to the treatment of cherry eye. What usually sparks this is that they are quoted around £200–300 for the surgical correction of this problem. Then they see on a Facebook forum or some other such place that actually you can get it done for about £60. This raises obvious questions in their minds. How dare one vet charge so much when it can clearly be done much less expensively? The answer is simple. The vet charging more is doing the correct procedure that is more beneficial to the animal

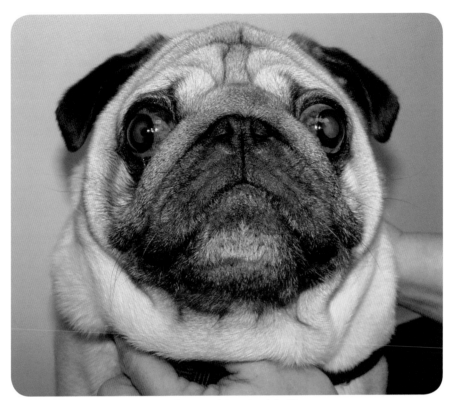

Figure 3.23: Facial skin folds can rub on bulging eyes. (Photo: David Gould)

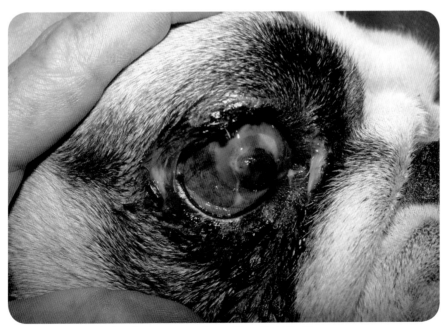

Figure 3.24: Some non-healing ulcers can rupture the eye. (Photo: David Gould)

and the other is pandering to owners and breeders by doing an outdated, simple snip that can cause lifelong problems in almost half the animals.

The correct way to treat cherry eye is to anaesthetise the animal and surgically replace the prolapsed gland. This means that this important, tear-producing gland can continue to provide an essential part of normal tear production. The quick fix of simply snipping the gland off makes it look fixed, but without this gland almost half of these dogs go on to get dry-eye later in life. This is a painful condition that can be difficult to treat and can cause further eye damage, ulceration and, in some cases, loss of the eye.

Some brachy breed websites tell owners specifically not to let their vet try to replace the gland and to just have it cut off. I'm sure you can understand how incredibly frustrating this is for the majority of the veterinary profession!

As you can see, the front end of these dogs and cats is markedly deformed and they have an unacceptably high level of disease caused by the shape of their head, a shape that we must always remember *we* have given them. For many though it doesn't stop there and so we need to look at the other impacts of their conformation or body shape.

Intestinal Problems

As we have denied our dogs the ability to breathe normally we have also produced unexpected knock-on effects elsewhere. We now know that brachycephalic dogs are more likely to suffer from a range of gastro-intestinal problems. Brachy dogs tend to swallow and gulp air in their efforts to breathe. Because it is difficult for some dogs to eat and breathe at the same time you see much higher levels of vomiting and regurgitation. As well as this the dogs experience very abnormal pressures in their chests when they breathe. Basically, the restricted airway translates into a huge effort to aid air intake. This negative pressure in the chest literally sucks part of their stomach through the diaphragm into the chest and causes hernias. It can also cause high rates of oesophageal reflux. This is where acids and juices from the stomach are forced up into the oesophagus, causing damage, ulcers and potentially severe problems, such as strictures. Studies have shown that even dogs not showing any intestinal signs often have lesions in their gastro-intestinal tract of which owners are unaware.

Spinal Problems

Some of the breed standards for these dogs call for curly or corkscrew tails; those short, stubby tails that are seen as so 'desirable' in the likes of pugs and bulldogs. As we said right at the beginning of the book, when you choose animals for breeding based solely on their appearance you unwittingly ignore their health. As we have selected for abnormally short or curly tails we have bred these animals to have spinal abnormalities called hemivertebrae. This is where the bones in the spine grow in an abnormal shape and make the spine twist. This is what produces the twisted tail, but it can also affect the rest of the spine, too. Some of these animals have pain during their early months when they are growing, but can also go on to lose the ability to walk or become incontinent. Surgery can help some but not all, and it's a major operation for any animal. It is surgery that could be prevented if we didn't 'need' that stubby, twisted tail ...

Passing the Basic Test

You may have noticed I mentioned big heads in an earlier subtitle. The level of disease and deformity in brachy animals is unquestionable, but one of the most damning facts about many of these breeds is their reproductive problems. Where breed standards call for large heads and narrow pelvises the natural outcome is puppies and kittens that do not fit through their mothers' pelvises. The level of Caesarean sections among many of these breeds is huge, with many matings needing assistance as well. It's important to remember that with their severely compromised airways these animals are also at a much higher risk from anaesthetic complications when they do require surgery, such as for Caesarean sections. One study found that about 85% of French bulldogs were born by C-section. That's nature's way of telling you something is terribly wrong with what you're doing.

A very wise person once said that if a group of animals can't pass the most basic test of reproduction then their continued existence must be closely scrutinised and questioned. Brachy animals are just clinging to existence through human intervention and it's time we accept that we made a mistake and we keep on making it.

The fact is that veterinary bodies from all over the world now urge people not to buy flat-faced dogs and cats. Many of the top medical and surgical specialists feel that the brachycephalic shape is completely unacceptable on welfare grounds. Sadly, our voice has made little impact because we can't get to people before they buy their puppy or kitten and fall in love. Social media posts and videos fan the flames of gross misunderstanding and the suffering of thousands of animals continues.

Not every brachy animal is severely affected by the things I've told you about, but the studies show that so many of them are that it is time to say *no more*. Do not under-estimate the suffering of these animals. As we said, more than one-half of owners of these dogs don't even recognise signs of respiratory distress in their animals because it is so normalised. Try putting a peg on your nose and breathing through a straw and see how long you can tolerate it before the panic sets in and you may have some idea of what a lifetime is like for these animals.

Please do not choose a flat-faced or undershot dog *or* cat. This body shape causes huge levels of unnecessary suffering in both species, and without veterinary intervention these breeds would simply disappear within a couple of generations because many are incompatible with life and reproduction. By making the decision not to buy or own these animals you will immediately improve your chances of getting a healthy pet and also vastly improve animal welfare in general.

In October 2017 I attended a two-day conference on inherited and conformational disease. World-leading vets from many specialities were there to give unquestionable expert opinion. I'll leave you with a quote from one that summed it all up for me:

'Brachycephaly is a direct result of the stupidity of man.'

Chapter 4

Short Legs, Long Backs and Bent Ears

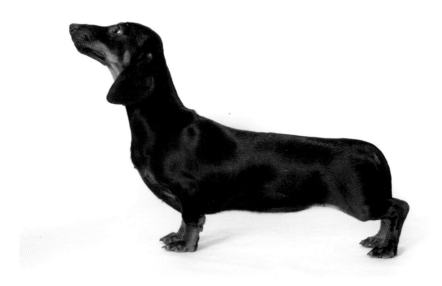

MANY OF OUR BREEDS OF DOG HAVE BODIES THAT ARE RELATIVELY long compared not only to the strength and size of the rest of the animal, but also to the length of the limbs. The problem with this is partly a matter of mechanics and engineering and partly one of genetic manipulation of growth. If you designed a bridge that had weak supports and a very long span it would fail without question. It is a fact that a long span must have support, either from the centre or from suspension. In these dogs the spine is the span of the bridge, but they have no support in the middle. The spine therefore is under an enormous amount of stress and can collapse. Many breeds have been 'engineered' this way, either with short legs, long back or both. Examples include the Jack Russell, bulldogs, basset family, Dandie Dinmont, Cesky terrier, Skye terrier, corgi and, most notably, for the combination of the two, the dachshund.

According to the Kennel Club book of breed standards from 2004, 'the length of the back and the character of the discs between the vertebrae of the spine have a tendency to allow a weakening in the area, and it is therefore important that the loin should be short and strong, and that individuals should not be allowed to become obese.'

The updated breed standard from the Kennel Club book 2017 says of the breed that the general appearance should be, 'Moderately long and low with no exaggeration, compact, well-muscled body, with enough ground clearance to allow free movement.' When you see photographs of dachshunds from a hundred years ago compared to the modern ones there is a striking difference in the length of the back and the shortness of the legs. The photographs of dachshunds in the updated breed standard book beggar belief. The dogs' legs are practically non-existent, their backs are super long and alarmingly, as with so many dogs these days, some of them are clearly overweight.

I always feel a very odd mixture of hilarity and absolute rage when I read breed standards. The fact that someone has actually had to state that a dog should ideally not scuff the ground when it walks really is ridiculous. When the KC writes the breed standards I always wonder if it ever takes a moment to ponder just how absurd some of them are.

What the breed standard book does not tell you is that dogs such as dachshunds and corgis are what we call 'chondrodystrophic' or 'achondroplastic'. These terms are a grand way of saying that the breeds cannot make cartilage properly. The trait is an inherited one and is similar to dwarfism in humans.

The 'weakening' that the Kennel Club book described is where changed and abnormal cartilage making up the discs in the spine fail over time. This can cause progressive or sudden paralysis. The cartilage fails all over the body to a degree, but it is most apparent in several areas of the back because of the stresses on the over-long back during normal movement. Many of these dogs require spinal surgery to have any hope of walking again and some have to be put to sleep because of the condition. So, effectively we have designed a long bridge not only with no supports, but with faulty materials, destined to fall into the abyss below.

The fact that this trait is inherited should come as no surprise because we have actually selected for it over time. To me, as with many of these conformational abnormalities that are now viewed as the norm, it should be unacceptable to deliberately breed a defect into an animal to provide a certain look.

Chondrodystrophic breeds have short, bowed limbs. The selection for shortened limbs probably started for a reason when dogs were used for hunting rabbits, badgers, rats and the like, and needed to be able to get down holes of various sizes. What has happened since, with the passage of time and the continued selection for extremes of these traits, is that the bones in the legs have become twisted and deformed. If you look at X-rays of the legs of breeds such as the dachshund and the basset, the bones are almost unrecognisable when compared to those of their distant ancestors and, of course, of modern, non-chondrodystrophic breeds. As the bones have become distorted the mechanical stresses and strains on the joints have changed. A 'normal', largely straight, limb has evolved over the centuries with muscle attachments in exactly the right places to achieve very efficient movement and maximum strength. Joints fit well together and healthy cartilage ensures smooth and even movement of the joints (see Figures 4.1–4.4).

In breeds with deformed legs and joints the muscles pull in an abnormal way and the joint surfaces can no longer meet as they are intended to do. This, in turn, can cause the early onset of arthritis or degenerative joint disease because the joints do not function properly, the protective cartilage becomes eroded and the shock-absorbing joint fluid becomes thin and watery.

The Kennel Club book 2004 tells us that bassets originated in France, where the term *basset* means short-leggedness. With a laughable sense of national pride, it also tells us that, although the basset originated in France, 'the breed was developed to perfection in Britain'. Hmm, we have managed to 'perfectly' develop one of the unhealthiest, ungainly and potentially unhappy breeds there is. The book also tells us that at only 38cm high at the shoulder, but weighing some 32 kilos, the dog is apparently 'quite difficult to pick up to put in a hatchback'. Perhaps we should be pondering whether legs this short and twisted are capable of comfortably carrying 32 kilos of weight and whether we should possibly expect a 'normal dog' to be able to get into a car unaided.

The new, 'healthy' breed standard book tells us of the breed's French origins, but doesn't mention it was us who ruined, sorry, perfected it. It says in the introduction to the breed that they originally were low to the ground with long fine ears to 'enclose the scent' of the prey and loose, elastic skin for protection (I'm not sure from what). We'll talk about these 'fine' ears and elastic skin later. The updated book makes a point of saying that these two functional features must not be exaggerated and the breed, 'should retain athletic fitness and good ground clearance to keep him fit for his original purpose'.

Now, it is clear that the KC is trying to make lots of noise in the updated breed standards about not breeding for exaggerated features and aiming for healthier specimens. While this is laudable the fact is that these dogs are so exaggerated already that it's too late. The words say one thing, but the photographs that accompany them are the exact opposite. If the pictures in *the* definitive guide to breed standards depict a basset with huge ears, clear exposure of the membranes of its eyes from the drooping skin, a heavy body, tiny, thick legs and a chest that appears to be about 3in off the ground, how are prospective owners or indeed breeders supposed to opt for something quite different? It's impossible.

Shortened legs, whether chondrodystrophoid or not, have also given rise to troubles such as luxating patellae (slipping knee caps). Many of the breeds with

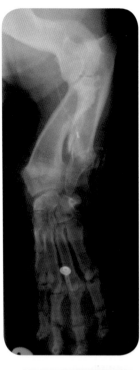

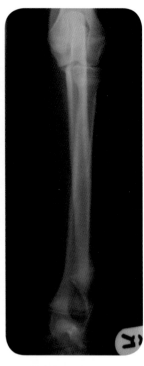

Figure 4.1 (top left): Front view basset foreleg. (Photo Andy Moores)

Figure 4.2 (top right): Front view normal foreleg. (Photo Andy Moores)

Figure 4.3 (bottom left): Side view normal foreleg. (Photo Andy Moores)

Figure 4.3 (bottom right): Side view basset foreleg. (Photo Andy Moores)

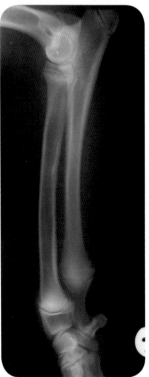

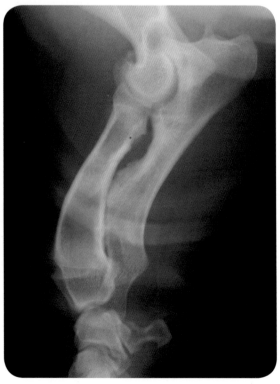

shortened legs, such as the terriers (particularly the Yorkshire terrier and Jack Russell), and others, including the miniature poodle, are extremely prone to this phenomenon. The reasons for luxation probably involve a number of factors. The most likely to play an early role is a misalignment of the major muscles and bones in the leg. The large group of muscles called the quadriceps on the front of the thigh is attached to the top of the tibia by a tendon in which the kneecap sits. These muscles are extremely strong and act to straighten the leg from a bent position. If the legs are slightly bowed this massive muscle group will effectively be trying to pull the kneecap out of the groove it sits in. In many of these breeds, probably as a result of inherited traits over time, this groove has become shallow or non-existent and so the muscles can pull the kneecap out of place almost constantly. It is also thought that in a circular way the pull of these muscle groups in young animals with bowed legs can deform the legs even more as they grow because the abnormal strains on the growth plates in the bones further distort the way they develop. There is a wide range of severity, but many require surgical intervention and nearly all will develop arthritis prematurely because of the joint instability and incongruity.

I once encountered an eight-week-old Yorkie puppy that came in for its first vaccination. The owners placed the dog and its sister on the table and it was immediately apparent that the male had something very wrong with him. He walked with his back legs completely straight and his spine had already become curved in an attempt to compensate for his dysfunctional back legs. I mentioned it to the owners and they said they had thought he wasn't quite right. They also told me that when they had gone to see the puppies the breeder had let all the other puppies run around on the floor, but had handed this one straight to them to hold. Now being the cynic that I am, I assumed that the breeder had noticed the deformity, which was quite striking, and was trying to fob them off. I may be wrong, but it seemed a big coincidence.

On examination I found that the back legs would not bend at all, so I said we would have to X-ray him. I sent the X-rays to an orthopaedic specialist to make sure I gave the owners the right advice. The report showed that the legs were so deformed that the patellae were so permanently luxated and small that they sat at the *back* of the knee. The dog was euthanased. Putting young animals to sleep is the worst part of my job. It is such a waste and in cases like this it is even more galling because it is so unnecessary. For me it is upsetting, but for the owners who have always already fallen head over heels in love with their puppies it is devastating.

As I mentioned in the early chapters, dogs' shapes have been changed way more than cats' over the years. Cats had one job to do and their shape suited them perfectly for it; we didn't need to meddle with them. Until the show world and breed standards came along, that is. As we mentioned with the flat-faced breeds

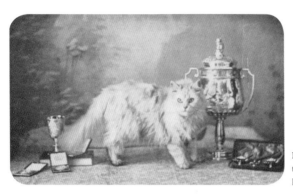

Figure 4.5: You'll be shocked to see that 100 years or so ago Persians looked like this! (Photo: Adobe Stock)

such as Persians, the very slightly shorter face of the 1900s is now unrecognisably flattened or even concave (see Figure 4.5).

Disastrously, people have now started to breed the cat equivalent of the dachshund. During the time I was writing the first book on pedigree issues I heard an interview with Paris Hilton that left me feeling very angry. She was describing how she is an enormous lover of animals (let's not talk about the captive monkeys) and during the list of her pets she disclosed that she had two (I think) Munchkin kittens. Steve Wright, who was interviewing her, asked what they were and she said they were cats that had all four legs very short, 'about two inches long', and they are 'like so cute'.

I drove home, got straight on the computer and was amazed. These cats were everywhere. According to Wikipedia, in 1983, Sandra Hochenedel, a music teacher in Louisiana, found two pregnant cats that had been chased by a bulldog under a truck. She kept one of the cats and named her Blackberry, and half of her kittens were born short-legged. Hochenedel gave a short-legged male kitten from one of Blackberry's litters to a friend, Kay LaFrance, and she named the kitten Toulouse. It is from Blackberry and Toulouse that today's Munchkin breed is descended. If this isn't the absolute epitome of inbreeding I don't know what is.

The Munchkin enthusiasts are quick to point out that the defect happens naturally and a few examples of short-legged cats have been reported in history. I don't know the exact number of normal cats there are in the world, but I would guess it is in the high millions, if not billions, so I'm guessing that a few lines (that have all naturally disappeared by the way, probably because they are incapable of climbing, hunting and running normally) doesn't really make it that 'normal'.

Since the breed appeared studies suggest that they are not truly chondrodystrophic like the dog breeds we mentioned. They don't seem to have the same spinal problems and have been found to have 'pseudoachondroplasia'. However, let's be quite clear that this is still a genetic defect that is being selected for. Although they don't seem to have the *same* issues as dogs they are still prone to curved spines and flattened chests as well as the short legs.

We always need to remember what nature intended for these animals. Munchkin cats can't climb properly and can struggle coming down stairs and so on, and many can't groom adequately. Their deformed limbs, just the same as in dogs, are prone to premature joint disease and many of these animals spend their lives in chronic pain. The brilliant welfare organisation, International Cat Care, is very clear when it comes to these issues and states quite clearly that they simply should not be bred.

The type of gene that gives the Munchkins their short legs is dominant. I won't go into the nitty gritty of genetics, but if you breed two short-legged Munchkins together a quarter of the kittens are likely to inherit a double dose of the gene. These kittens never survive and die before birth. Half the remaining kittens are likely to be short-legged and a quarter could be normal. These types of animals are not perpetuated by nature because nature selects for healthy animals, fit for purpose. Munchkin cats are not. Do not buy one.

Sadly, the breed is now recognised by several large cat organisations and is also shown, has a breed standard and is fast gaining in popularity. I find this soul-destroying and actually think it should be illegal to breed animals based on a severely debilitating health problem.

I'm a little surprised in this age of political correctness that no one seems to think it even slightly inappropriate to have named a whole breed after the vertically challenged characters from the *Wizard of Oz* played by actors with dwarfism.

The bent ears in the title of this chapter refer to another breed of cat in which we have selected for abnormal cartilage to give a certain look – the Scottish fold. Scottish fold cats are popular with some because their bent ears give them a 'cute' baby face. Once more we come back to our wish for human baby characteristics in our pet animals.

As with the dramatic inbreeding of the Munchkin breed, this breed can be traced back to one female cat in 1961. She had bent ears and had a litter of kittens, some of which had bent ears. A neighbour who was a 'cat fancier', or deformity lover may be more appropriate in this case, took one of the kittens and the breed began.

The ears of the Scottish fold bend forward because the cartilage is defective. Of course, you don't get defective cartilage in just one area; exactly the same as with our chondrodystrophic dogs, the cartilage all over the body is affected.

The cats are born with straight ears, but they become folded during the first few weeks of life. As with so much insane human manipulation of nature's accidents, breeders have 'excelled' themselves and managed to create cats with double or triple folds so that the ears lay almost flat on the head. The round face, flat ears and wide eyes give them an owl-like appearance. The only thing is that owls evolved by natural selection and survival of the fittest, not through selection for disease.

The defect that gives the bent ears causes crippling joint disease elsewhere in the body and although there is a wide variation in severity it is a significant health concern in these animals. The Governing Council of the Cat Fancy (GCCF), which is the cat equivalent of the KC, did recognise the breed in the 1960s, but in 1971 revoked this because of the devastating level of joint disease. Lovers of the breed claim that by only mating folds to normal cats you can keep the disease to a minimum and have unaffected cats that still have the folded ears.

On the other side of the pond, the Cat Fancier's Association, a US equivalent of the GCCF, has this to say about the breed, 'Scottish Fold kittens are born with straight ears. At about three to four weeks of age, their ears fold … or they don't! It is usually around 11 to 12 weeks of age that the breeder can determine the quality (pet, breeder or show). Presently, only folded ear cats of Scottish lineage are permitted in the show ring, and naturally, every breeder wants to produce show cats.' This is another classic example of an unquestionably, detrimental genetic defect being selected for, for the show ring. It is simply indefensible. Notice that presumably the poorer quality cats are the ones selected to be pets. Shouldn't we be aiming for all our pet and show animals to be able to expect as healthy and pain free a life as possible?

Astonishingly, amidst all the information elsewhere and concern about the crippling arthritis in this breed the CFA goes on to say, 'Scottish Folds are hardy cats, much like their barnyard ancestors … The Scottish Fold is an undemanding cat. A clean environment, proper nutrition, and generous doses of love are its only requirements.' On the whole breed page on the CFA website there is not a single mention of the fact that the ears are bent due to a cartilage defect. No mention of joint problems or the fact that many of these cats spend their lives under veterinary care in an attempt to manage their pain. Somehow I doubt that love and good food are this breed's only requirements.

Despite this there are many welfare and veterinary organisations who feel, like I do, that we simply should not be breeding them at all. No matter how small the number of cats eventually affected they could all be avoided by not selecting for a gene that causes disease. Cat lovers should love cats as nature intended.

Trying to keep breeds alive through manipulation and veterinary intervention is just not acceptable. Dogs have suffered for hundreds of years and I am desperately sad that it seems to be going the same way for cats. We need to stop the demand right now for breeds whose very standards rely on genetic deformity and disease.

Just before you go to the next chapter, here is a reminder of what natural animals look like compared to man's creations …

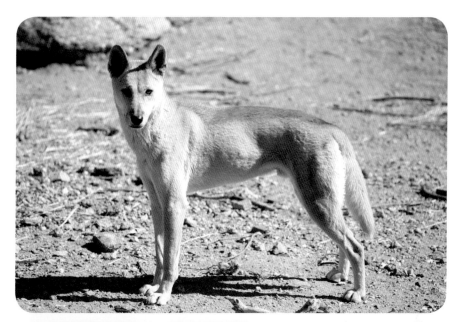

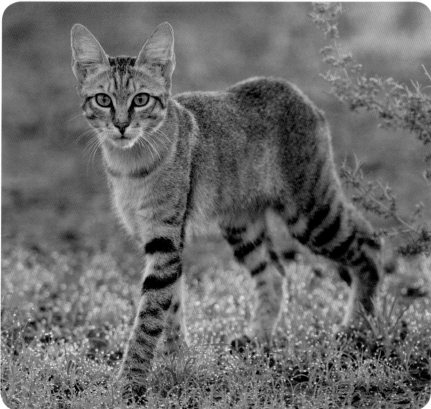

Figures 4.6, 4.7: Natural canids and felids have long, straight legs. (Photo: Adobe Stock)

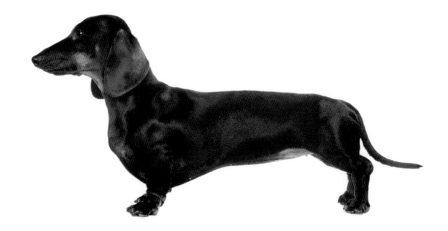

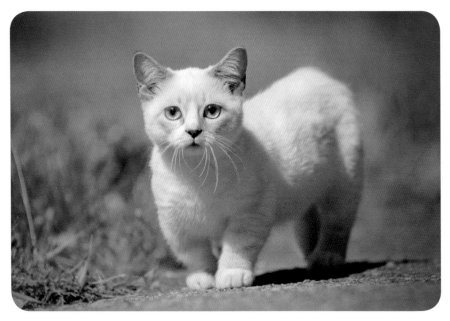

Figures 4.8, 4.9: We have effectively amputated the legs of some dog and cat breeds. (Photo: Adobe Stock)

Chapter 5

Slip Me Some Skin!

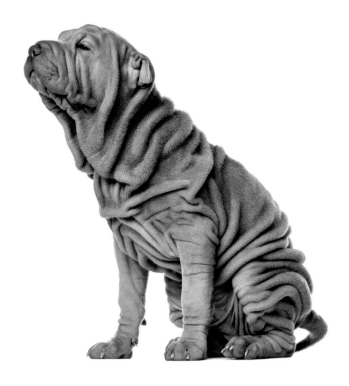

A S I MENTIONED IN PASSING IN THE PREVIOUS CHAPTERS, ONE FEATURE that usually goes hand in hand with short legs, and indeed short faces, is skin folds. As we have shortened skulls and legs the skin has not shortened with them in some breeds. Therefore you have the same amount of skin, but just bunched up like a wrinkled sock. Now, strangely, skin folds are something that many people find cute. You see a poster of a wrinkly boxer or bulldog puppy or, even worse, a Shar-Pei and everyone starts swooning over how cute they are. It is not until you have seen the horribly inflamed and chronically infected skin that sits in between these folds that you start to revise your opinion. Skin is not designed to be permanently folded; you will not find examples of it anywhere in nature. Yes, animals such as rhinos and elephants have wrinkles, but these open up as the animal moves, they live in very dry places and their skin is not covered in fur. In people that are extremely obese we see the same infected folds between the rolls of fat. I'm sure anyone that has suffered with it will tell you how unpleasant it is.

The skin is the largest organ in the body, and our skin and that of all animals is amazing. Skin can clean itself, it is waterproof and it supports an incredible number of bacteria. These bacteria in general are in balance; they live in their own little microclimate and, as long as the skin remains unbroken, don't usually cause any problems. When you fold a piece of skin you alter that climate; you make it warm and moist and you stop the air getting to it. This causes some bacteria that thrive in air to die and it lets a lot of other bacteria grow and reproduce in vast numbers.

Normal skin has a fine balance of oils and nutrients that keep it healthy. Once the skin is folded it becomes moist and this constant moisture starts to soften and weaken the skin; bacteria then start to get into the top layers and the body mounts a response to try to kill them. This is inflammation. The skin becomes inflamed, infected and intensely itchy and red. Dogs with skin-fold pyoderma (skin infection) are depressing cases. They often need repeated courses of antibiotics and they very rarely get better without surgical removal of the offending folds. Some people joke about these dogs having to have 'facelifts'. While it may be humorous to mock the latest celebrity that has gone under the knife for the sake of vanity, having to give dogs anaesthetics and surgery simply to make life bearable doesn't seem very funny to me.

When I looked through the UK breed standards I counted more than 20 breeds in which having wrinkles or a dewlap, which is basically a giant neck skin fold, is either part of the breed standard, so desirable, or clearly visible on the photographs in the book. Interestingly, the standard for the Boston terrier clearly states that the skull and the muzzle should be free from wrinkles, but both the photographs show skin folds on the face; and non-existent nostrils, obviously.

In many breeds loose skin is seen as desirable, like the basset we mentioned, but also breeds such as the bloodhound and the mastiffs. The big droopy face is another excess of skin and all the breeds with dewlaps will also be prone to abnormal skin fold problems. Many of the breeds with drooping lips will tend to slobber and drool because the lips are abnormal and don't function properly. This constant saliva under the neck can also add to the damp conditions.

A few years after qualifying, when I was on television a lot, I was asked to go to Crufts to be on a stand and sign autographs. I went and vowed I would never go back. However, in 2017, the wonderful people working tirelessly to improve the health of Cavalier spaniels asked if I would go with them to present the Kennel Club with a petition signed by more than 30,000 like-minded people. I broke my vow and headed back into my idea of hell. While we were there we encountered a couple with a St Bernard, a breed in which the standard calls for a well-developed dewlap. Lots of people were laughing and stopping to take photographs of the dog because it had a 'hilarious' bib on that said, 'Love me, love my drool.' The couple seemed quite proud of it.

I asked if I could take a photo (for quite different reasons) and as I snapped away the dog raised its head. The whole of its dewlap was an inflamed and clearly diseased mass of sore skin. Not really anything to be proud of or boast about.

The Dogue de Bordeaux and the Neapolitan mastiff are some of the worst affected by the breed standard need for loose skin or wrinkles. The updated standards make a point of saying that for the Neapolitan the loose skin should not be excessive and that the wrinkles on the face of the Dogue de Bordeaux should be 'fine'. Now, I don't think it's just me, but when you look at Figure 5.1 and 5.2 maybe you can be the judge of whether the Neapolitan is excessive or the wrinkles on the DDB are fine. To my mind fine wrinkles are like crow's feet or laughter lines, not these dogs' faces.

Dogs with droopy, skin-laden heads and faces tend to have something we call 'diamond eye' (see Figures 5.3 and 5.4). This is where their eyes are affected by conditions called entropion and ectropion at the same time. Entropion is where an eyelid rolls inwards and the eyelashes constantly rub against the eye itself. It is a very painful condition and leads to corneal ulcers, self-trauma and sometimes the loss of the eye. Ectropion is the opposite and is where an eyelid rolls away from the eye. This isn't always a medical problem but does expose the eye, so may make it drier than a normal eye and can also lead to tears spilling over on to the face because of the drooping lid.

In dogs with diamond eye they tend to have entropion of the upper lids because of the heavy skin on top of the head and brow and ectropion of the bottom lid where the weight of the skin underneath drags the eyelid away from the eye. Many cartoon bassets and bloodhounds have these characteristic droopy, red eyes, but in reality the condition is nothing to be celebrated. Some of the most difficult diamond eyes to correct are those where one eyelid, usually the top one, has both conditions in different areas. Most cases of entropion in adulthood will require surgical correction to try to relieve the pain and stop the trauma to the eyes. Sadly, if you Google diamond eye in dogs you are immediately presented with an abundance of products to helpfully remove the tear staining caused by the tear overflow. None of this would be necessary if we were not selecting for deformity.

When I worked in York my husband had to operate on an absolutely dreadful Neapolitan. The poor creature had already lost the sight in one eye from the damage from the eyelids and the other was chronically scarred. The dog had to have a huge swathe of skin the size of a dinner plate removed from the top of his head in order to pull the skin of the face upwards and allow correction of the eyelids. This is certainly not an isolated case.

Eyes can also become damaged by skin, as we said with the brachys, where the

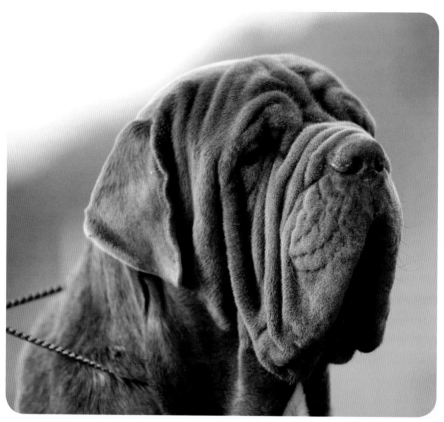

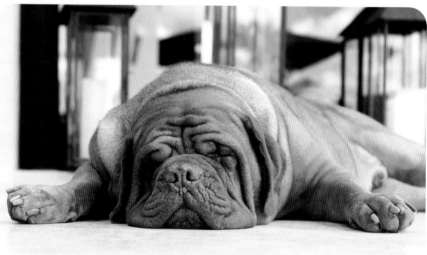

Figures 5.1, 5.2: More than fine wrinkles. (Photo: Adobe Stock)

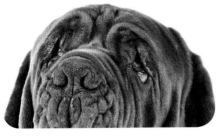
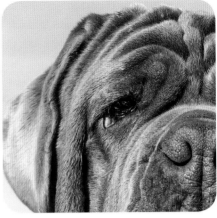

Figures 5.3, 5.4: Diamond eye: the top lid rolls inwards under the heavy brow, the bottom lid is dragged away by the weight of the facial skin. (Photo: Adobe Stock)

skin folds on the shortened nose actually impinge on the bulging eyes. Surgery is often needed in these cases to remove the skin fold, which sadly some breeders are opposed to because it ruins the desired look.

Over the years when I have been a little vocal about issues like this I have encountered some quite bizarre retorts. I once pointed out that a show-winning, white bulldog quite clearly had skin-fold pyoderma because you could see the red, inflamed patches against the white of the face. The dog's eyes were barely open and it looked in clear discomfort, possibly from entropion. It never should have been admitted to a show, let alone be winning best of breed.

When I pointed this out in an article I was writing about brachycephaly I received a torrent of abuse and vitriol from owners and breeders of bulldogs. Many of them rather oddly went to great lengths to tell me about how much attention they gave to the daily care of the facial folds of their dogs, as if this was a really good thing. One woman told me crossly that her dog's daily skin care regime was even better than hers. They had all quite clearly missed the point. Since I was 11 years old I've owned three, canid-shaped cross-breeds and five moggie cats. I have never, ever had to clean their face or devote any time to a 'skin-care' regime for them. Normal animals do not need daily washes, creams and routines because their skin is not wrinkled and they are healthy.

Can you imagine if a dingo, wolf or tiger had chronically infected patches of skin? They would self-traumatise, get deeper and deeper infections followed by generalised septicaemia and then die. They would not pass on their genes. If they didn't die quickly their constant discomfort and inflammation would make it more difficult to hunt, the infected skin would attract insects and maggots and the inevitable end would still come, but just very slowly.

Perhaps the epitome of all skin disease breeds is the Shar-Pei. They originate from China and were used as fighting and hunting dogs. Originally they had slightly loose skin to allow them to get some protection if they were grabbed in a fight. As with all our extremes, this was taken to ridiculous lengths by breeders in the last few decades until the dogs look like someone has stretched their skin on a rack and then put it back on. Tragically these 'cute', wrinkly puppies and adults have been used time and again for skin care adverts for humans. 'Want younger looking skin?' they say with a picture of a firm-skinned, Photoshopped woman cuddling a wrinkled, deformed and diseased puppy. None of this is OK!

A huge percentage of Shar-Peis suffered from entropion because of the appalling excess of skin and heavy wrinkles on their faces. The Kennel Club book of 2004 tells us that this had already been addressed by breeders even then. The prevalence may well be falling, but vets are still seeing these dogs for multiple reasons, continued entropion being one of them.

The breed standard in 2004, under the characteristics heading, said, 'Loose skin, frowning expression, harsh bristly coat'. As I've said, the updated standards of 2017 are extolled by the Kennel Club as being much less exaggerated and therefore providing guidance for breeders to breed much healthier, less exaggerated animals. In the 2017 Shar-Pei standard the characteristics section says, 'Relatively loose skin, frowning expression, harsh bristly coat.'

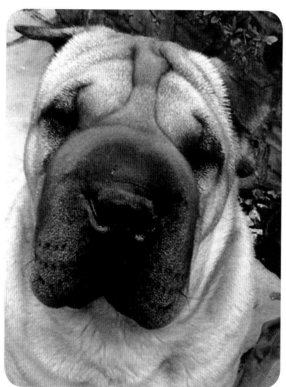

Figure 5.5: Entropion and padding.
(Photo: Tanya Banks)

Oh I see, the word 'relatively' makes that a much healthier dog! Note that they still demand a frowning expression, which translates as heavy wrinkles on the head and face. In fact, the more exact wording later in the standard has changed from 'fine wrinkles' in 2004 to 'moderate wrinkles' in 2017. I'm struggling to see how that is better, but the dogs pictured in both books have what I would call more than moderate wrinkles.

One of the very distinctive characteristics of the Shar-Pei is the 'padded' lips and muzzle. I use this word because that's what the breed standard demands and calls it. In 2004 the standard said, 'The lips and top of muzzle padded, causing a slight bulge at the base of the nose. When viewed from front, bottom jaw appears wider than top due to padding of lips.'

The revised standard says this, 'The lips and top of muzzle may be slightly padded. When viewed from front, bottom jaw appears wider than top.' This is clearly still saying that the reason the bottom jaw appears wider than the top is because of the padding. You may be wondering why I'm so hung up on the padding. It's because it is an inherited defect in the skin that is specifically being selected for.

The deep genetics of it and the problem itself are way beyond my medical understanding, but the effects of this defect are clear to any vet who has ever been presented with a Shar-Pei. The defect means the dog's skin is generally inflamed and abnormal, and it is this variation in swelling and inflammation that causes the desired 'padding'. The problem also makes the dogs more prone to inflammatory reactions in general, can contribute to Shar-Pei fevers and also a condition called amyloidosis that can lead to liver and kidney failure. And all this because they are 'supposed' to have padded faces. Every small animal vet will have seen the appalling skin disease, infections and inflammation that these dogs get due to this condition combined with their wrinkles. On top of this, the closely folded, thickened ears can't drain properly, have diseased skin inside and out and are a frequent cause of otitis (inflamed ears), infections and chronic pain in many dogs. It is totally unacceptable to breed for this abnormality.

A friend of mine who is a vet ended up advising some anti-inflammatories for a Shar-Pei for an unrelated problem and when he did the follow-up consultation the dog had recovered beautifully. However, the owner had complained because all the swelling in the dog's head had gone away and it 'didn't look like a Shar-Pei anymore'. Maybe this owner should have stopped to ask him or herself whether the dog would prefer not to look like a Shar-Pei and actually have comfortable skin.

You can test for this abnormality, and thankfully some breeders are, but when you compare any of the Western wrinkled versions of this breed with the original type they are virtually unrecognisable as the same breed. The only way we will eliminate the inflammatory diseases from Shar-Peis is if we decide we don't need them to have wrinkles and padding anymore!

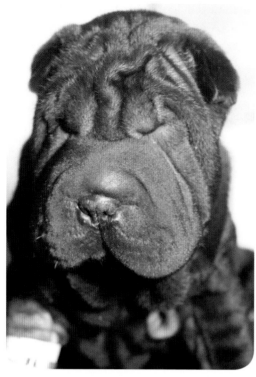

Figure 5.6: Severe entropion in a Shar-Pei puppy. (Photo: Dr David Gould)

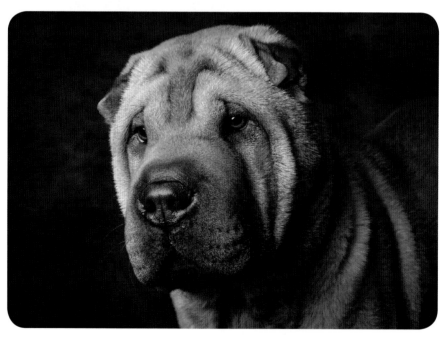

Figure 5.7: Even in Shar-Peis with better eyes the folded ears and padding are still abnormalities. (Photo: Adobe Stock)

When I was taught dermatology at university one of the first things the lecturer said has always stayed with me and I've since said it to many owners, 'Skin disease is one of the hardest things to manage. It is difficult to diagnose the cause, it can be difficult to treat and it never goes away, so is a lifelong problem.'

Most vets will have dealt with the obvious frustration of owners during the work-up of skin cases. These cases can be soul-destroying for the vet and the owner, they can undoubtedly cause long-term suffering for the patients and they can be very expensive. Getting to the bottom of skin disease can be a lengthy process of ruling things out. Inherited skin disease comes in many forms; some are due to skin conformation, such as the fold issues we discussed, and some, like the Shar-Pei, are because of a specific genetic defect; however, a growing problem now is atopic dermatitis.

Atopy, as it's also known, is seen much more in certain breeds of dogs than others, so although the exact inheritance isn't known it seems reasonable to assume there is an inherited factor to it. It is most commonly seen in breeds such as the Shar-Pei, wirehaired fox terrier, golden retriever, Dalmatian, boxer, Boston Terrier, Labrador retriever, Lhasa apso, Scottish terrier, shih-tzu, and West Highland white terrier.

Westies are hopefully improving through selective breeding for the better, but in the ten years or so after I qualified we used to see depressing numbers of these dogs. Their chronic itching and repeated trauma would often cause their skin to become thickened and black and they were referred to as 'armadillo Westies'. It isn't unheard of to hear about some animals with intractable skin diseases such as this being put to sleep at a young age because the owner felt the dog was suffering too much.

Atopy is an allergic reaction to environmental things such as grasses, pollens, house dust mites and fleas. You do see it in cats, but it is much more common in dogs, possibly (and this is me speculating) because pedigree dogs are so much more common than pedigree cats so the few cases we do see in cats are the odd one-offs you find in a large population.

Some dogs are allergic to one or two things and some seem to be sensitive to everything. It usually starts in young animals between the age of six months and about three years. It causes intense itching and the animals often cause self-trauma, which leads to infections and inflammation and long-term problems. For many dogs and their owners the level of itching and scratching is simply unbearable.

I used the word depressing earlier and these can be very depressing cases for everyone concerned, most of all the dog. If you do consider getting a pedigree dog, investigate their skin diseases and the family history very carefully. It could save you a lot of heartache and money.

To finish, here's a reminder of what nature chooses for skin on the head and round the eyes compared with what some breed standards choose.

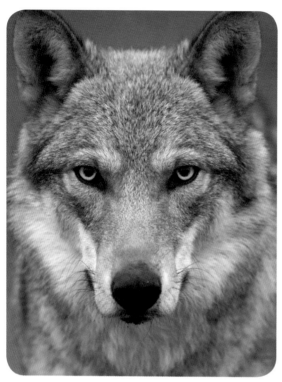

Figure 5.8: What nature intended ...
(Photo: Adobe Stock)

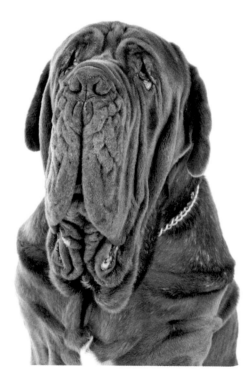

Figure 5.9: ... vs what man has done.
(Photo: Adobe Stock)

Chapter 6

Dumbo Dogs

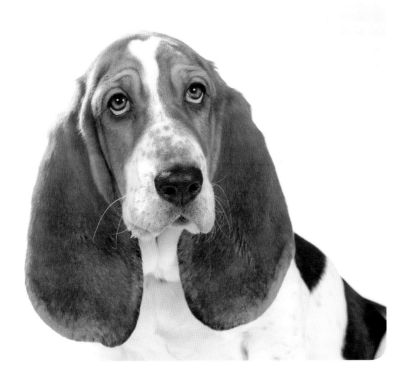

WHEN I WAS A CHILD I WAS MERCILESSLY RIDICULED FOR MY BIG ears. Dumbo, taxi with the doors open, the FA Cup, you name it; if there was an analogy for sticky out ears, I was called it. It wasn't much fun, but as there was nothing I could do about it I just had to get on with it, a kind of 'that which does not kill us makes us stronger' scenario.

With that history in mind maybe I shouldn't really start criticising those with large ears. The fact is though that my ears are a natural variation of a working organ and they still work perfectly even though they were the bane of my life for a while.

Sadly for our dogs, many of the ears that years of man-made selection has given them are far from natural and can cause great suffering. Many breeds have been bred to have ears that are heavy, hairy, long, thick and all variations in between. Wild canids and felids have upright, pricked, open ears. This allows them to hear extremely well and locate the source of a sound. The movement and position of the ears is also used as a form of communication. The insides of their ear canals are almost totally fur-free, having just a few sensitive hairs to trap dirt and dust. In these ears air can easily circulate. The canals are open allowing wax and debris from the canal to be expelled.

I'm sure you can see where I'm going with this. Owing to our desire for variations in ear shape and conformation we have taken a well-designed organ and made it malfunction. Although the actual hearing may not be directly affected there are many consequences of abnormal ear shape. I will give you some examples.

Basset hounds are the kings and queens of ridiculous ears (see Figure 6.1). The 2004 breed standard said the ears 'should' be 'Set on low, just below line of eye. Long; reaching well beyond end of muzzle of correct length, but not excessively so.' Laughably the new standards say '... reaching only slightly beyond end of muzzle ... but not excessively so.'

I'm not sure I understand this correctly. How can an ear that either reaches well beyond or even slightly beyond the length of the muzzle not be considered excessive? Either way, the ears should, according to the breed standard, touch and drag on the ground when the dog's head is lowered. Can you imagine an animal in nature having structures as sensitive as their ears dragging on the floor and being exposed to possible trauma? Of course not.

As well as the possible damage, most likely from being trodden on by the dog itself, the weight of the ear stops air getting into the canal and wax and debris getting

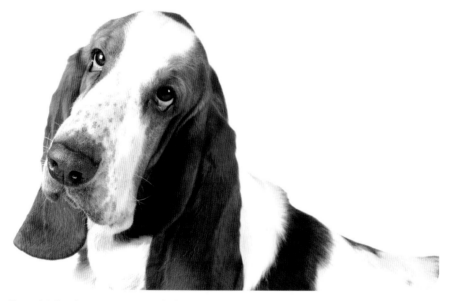

Figure 6.1: Ears that can trip you up are far from ideal! (Photo: Adobe Stock)

out. The canal will be moist and warm, and start to resemble all their other skin folds. Chronic infections are commonplace and sometimes, once again, surgical intervention may be necessary.

The nature of these ears also makes any surgery that's required more difficult. The ears have to be bandaged up on top of the head or 'pegged' together somehow. People think it very humorous post-operatively, but surgically they can be a nightmare. Many people will have fond memories of the Fred Basset cartoons, but when real animals start to resemble cartoons we need to start asking ourselves some serious ethical questions. (see Figure 6.2 and 6.3)

Bassets may be the worst affected by the size of their ears, but there are several other breeds trailing not far behind. Most of the other basset breeds, bloodhounds, dachshunds, all the setters and the pointers to name but a few, and then of course you have the spaniels.

Spaniels such as the Springer and the Cocker have very heavy, hairy ears and ear canals. I have spent numerous summers fishing grass seeds and twigs out of spaniels' ear canals. It seems strange that some people are very happy to pre-emptively amputate their tails in case of injury, but yet their ears should be 'long', 'extending to nose tip', 'fairly large', 'well clothed with long … hair', 'thick' and 'set low', depending on what particular spaniel they are. We'll talk about tail docking later, but I'd like to tell a little story here.

I try to live life by the no regrets rule. I try to have the philosophy that you

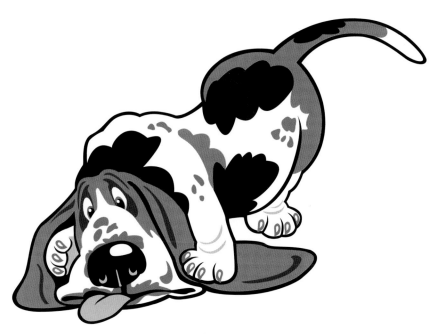

Figure 6.2: Cartoon basset. (Illustration: Adobe Stock)

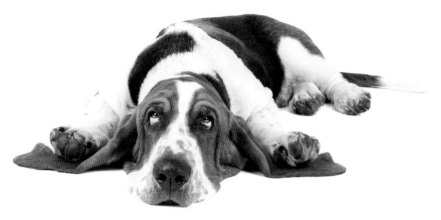

Figure 6.3: Actual basset. (Photo: Adobe Stock)

shouldn't regret things you've done because they are all experiences and part of our lifelong learning curve. However, there is one huge regret I have and that is from *not* doing something. During the time that I was working on the campaign to get the awful business of tail docking banned there was a picture endlessly circulated by the pro-docking lobby to try to illustrate why they thought tails should be indiscriminately cut off at birth.

The postcard propaganda showed a sweet-looking spaniel, fresh from the field, wet from the bushes and absolutely covered in blood from an injury to its tail. Any vet will tell you that the smallest cuts in tails bleed quickly, but once the tail has wagged about and the dog is wet they soon look like a crime scene when in fact they have only lost a few millilitres of blood. The photograph was designed to be shocking and I suspect the dog had a very minor cut. My regret is that during the time of the campaign I was also presented with an almost identical looking spaniel, wet from the field and covered in blood. The dog even sat, leaned against the consulting room wall in exactly the same pose. It had a cut in its pendulous ear, another area that bleeds profusely from minor cuts. I didn't have time to go and find the practice digital camera and it was before the days of cameras on mobile phones, so I never got my retaliatory snap. No spaniel lovers as far as I know are advocating a return to ear cropping. I've worked mainly in rural areas in practice where gundogs abound and the frequency of anaesthetics and surgery for ear trauma and foreign bodies is pretty high. But hey, we have to follow the breed standard!

We once dog-sat for a friend's working Springer, Henry. He is a very sweet dog with not a bad bone in his body and likes to think he is attached to you by a small piece of elastic that does not allow him to be further than a foot away from you at any time. We went to the woods with our dogs, 'the boys', where they love to be, and had our usual hour-long walk. Henry had a great time. He was doing what spaniels do best: rummaging and foraging around and generally tearing about like the proverbial headless chicken. His nose was glued to the floor. What astounded me was that his ears trailed constantly on the floor. We got back and they were absolutely covered in sticky buds and all sorts of woodland debris. I know our friend spends lots of time after every walk picking things out of Henry's ears and the covering fur, but I can't believe that large shooting estates can have the time to devote to this for their dogs. I know lots of people love spaniels, but surely some owners must admit that maybe it would be nice if their ears were just a bit *smaller*?

Poodles, among other breeds, have ear canals that are absolutely stuffed full of hair. This has the effect of reducing air flow and of trapping all the normal secretions of the ear lining in the canal. Again, chronic irritation and infection are commonplace. Some poodles need to have their ears plucked while at the grooming parlour. For those of you with that middle-aged phenomenon of hair in your ears, try pulling it out with tweezers and see what it feels like, then imagine hair extending right to your eardrum and see whether you would relish letting someone remove it by plucking! For the dogs that can't tolerate it conscious it means more unnecessary sedations and anaesthetics. I say unnecessary not because the vets shouldn't do it, the dogs are suffering after all, but because they simply should not have been bred this way.

As I said with skin disease, ear disease often arises out of a number of factors. Long gone are the days of saying dogs had 'canker'. In years gone by, ear disease was viewed mostly as an entity separate to the rest of the skin. Nowadays, however, we know that ear and skin disease are inextricably linked in some cases. After all, ears are covered in skin. Many breeds such as the basset, retriever, Labrador, Westie and poodle are prone to chronic ear disease, partly because of conformation in some cases and partly because of inherited or predisposed disease. My day list every summer used to be full of these dogs that were shaking their heads, scratching their ears and often traumatised because of the discomfort. Ask any vet what the most distinctive smells of our career are and somewhere on most people's list among the infected teeth, the anal glands and the rotting bovine placentas will be that grim, waxy, greasy smell that emanates from many of these dogs' ears.

Let's not forget the breeds with tightly folded ears as well, the Shar-Pei again, but also think back to the fold cats. Both cats and dogs have been made to have ears that are the opposite of what nature selects for.

I know we are all used to these breeds, but we have to start to look at them for what they are. It's not to say the dog inside that body is horrible or bad, but the shapes we've dealt them are. You would never find these ears in nature because they cause suffering, infections and make it harder to communicate and hear. These

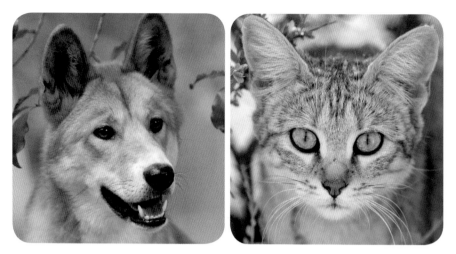

Figures 6.4, 6.5: Natural ears are erect, mobile and open. (Photo: Adobe Stock)

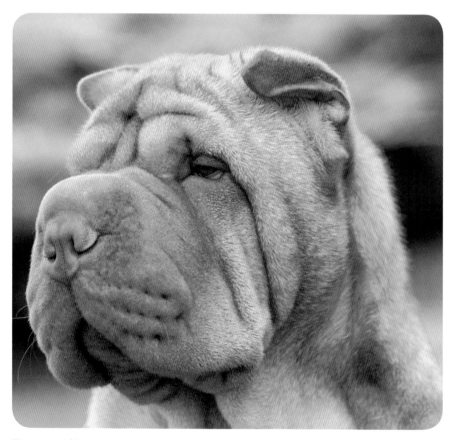

Figures 6.6: Folded ears are totally unnatural. (Photo: Adobe Stock; Shutterstock)

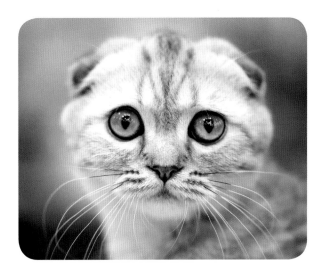

Figures 6.7: Folded ears are totally unnatural. (Photo: Adobe Stock)

ears would never naturally come about because of genetic diversity and natural selection for *health* not appearance. Many mongrel domestic dogs these days have ears that half flop over. On the whole these ears work, they can be pricked to communicate and locate sounds, they are usually still hair free inside and are in proportion with the dog's head. When you look for your puppy or kitten try to pick an individual or breed with moderate, open, clear ears that are closer to what Mother Nature intended.

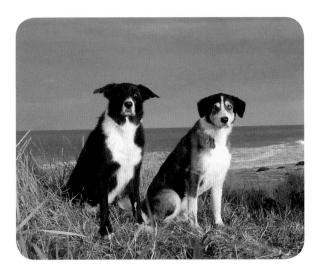

Figure 6.8: Pan and Badger sporting their various versions of proportioned, healthy ears!

Chapter 7

Tail Docking

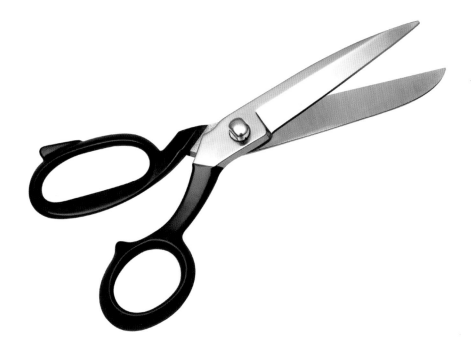

AS I MENTIONED MY LITTLE TAIL VERSUS EARS ANECDOTE IN THE LAST chapter, it seems sensible to talk about tail docking now. I had hoped that ten years on from the last book I wouldn't be including this chapter, but sadly tail docking does still go on and if you are reading this in one of many other countries it is still a very relevant thing to talk about. I was going to call this chapter simply 'Mutilations', which will give you a heads up about my feelings on the subject! For those of you that are uninitiated, you will either be angered, enlightened or both.

Big advances were made in the UK when it comes to tail docking when the Animal Welfare Act of 2006 came into force. Those of us who campaigned hard to get rid of tail docking altogether had hoped for an outright ban across the board for all breeds; there are no arguments to defend the practice after all. Sadly the vocal minority, my cynical side might say the rich landowners that some politicians like to keep sweet, managed to snatch it away at the last minute. The law varies from country to country, but many breeds of working dogs are exempt and can still have a healthy appendage amputated for no clinical reason whatsoever.

It is because of these exemptions, and because of all the countries in the world where it does go on, I still feel it is worth looking at what exactly it is and why some people believe it should continue.

For those of you that don't know, tail docking is when the tail of a puppy is removed between one and five days of age (although I know personally of one vet who carried it out at eight days of age because the breeder had been too busy and had forgotten to get it done). The tails are usually either cut off with scissors or a scalpel, or have a rubber band placed round them until the dead bit falls off. Now you will be told that, when carried out properly, this is a completely painless procedure. Indeed, the Council for Docked Breeds (CDB) maintains that some puppies docked while they are asleep will not even wake up. Let me ask you this; can you imagine a human baby sleeping peacefully through someone cutting off its little finger with a pair of scissors? Try putting a rubber band on the end of your finger and see how long it takes before the pain starts and then see how long you can stand it. I have personally spoken to many people, mostly unwilling nurses forced to hold the puppies, that have seen the procedure. I have yet to meet someone who was not sickened. I know that more than one of them threatened to resign if she was ever involved again. One vet I spoke to said that she used to insist the owners held their own puppies while it was done and a great many of them stopped asking for it to be done after that.

The fact is that the majority of people, when informed about the practice, are against the procedure and it is, in fact, only a small minority of showers, breeders and gundog owners that want it to continue. The fact is that there is still a massive amount of ignorance about it. I don't mean this in an offensive way. How can we expect the public to know the truth when the people who are docking these animals are so underhand about it? I was once told of someone who had been informed by a breeder of Jack Russells that 70% of them are born without tails now because they have been docked for so many years. This is evolutionary nonsense and is typical of the rubbish that is spoken by some of these people.

So, let's look at what the Council for Docked Breeds (CDB) says. Let's take each of its reasons for docking one by one and see what we think. It's not rocket science to pick them apart because not one of them has any logic behind it.

1. To Avoid Tail Damage

This is their favourite one. Many breeds of dogs have traditionally been docked to prevent tail damage later in life. Typically these have been working breeds, such as spaniels and pointers. Apparently their 'enthusiastic' tail action causes them untold misery and injury when they work. The CDB even goes on to suggest that for some dogs this injury 'can even happen in the home to non-working breeds'. Oh the horror!

Where do I begin? I have received lots of correspondence from owners of working undocked dogs that have never had a problem in their lives. As we said in the last chapter, why have spaniels been bred to have long, floppy, hairy ears when surely this is the first point of contact they have with gorse and brambles?

During the tail docking debate for the Animal Welfare Bill I heard many pro-docking people saying that if dogs had to be docked later in life due to injury they would have to undergo an anaesthetic and a prolonged and painful recovery. This is hypocritical nonsense. Firstly, they don't seem to be so concerned about the anaesthesia required for grass seed removal and ear injury surgery. Secondly, any surgical procedure should be pain-free due to the standard use of analgesics and, thirdly, within a week to ten days the tail is healed. If dogs aren't allowed sufficient time off work to recover from any surgery it is surely a cause for concern.

One breed we see very commonly used for working is the Labrador. Labradors have an incredibly 'waggy' tail and we do sometimes see a condition called 'Labrador tail' or 'swimmer's tail'. This is where the dog loses the ability to lift or move the tail, and it can be quite painful. It is generally considered to be fatigue from a day of strenuous wagging or swimming. Surely docking would prevent this terrible suffering? Oh no, that's right, Labradors aren't 'traditionally' docked.

In the case of pointers, I am even more at a loss. The English pointer is undocked, but the German pointer is docked. Even more odd is that the German shorthaired pointer is docked, but the German longhaired pointer is not! Why on earth are fox hounds not docked? The most important point to make here is that, as outlined by the RCVS, it is impossible to know at one to five days of age which dogs will be workers and which will be pets, so the injury argument is therefore not a valid reason for docking. Many of the terrier breeds were originally docked because of their work in confined spaces. Let me ask you this: when was the last time you saw a working Yorkshire terrier?

As for non-working breeds, the injury argument reaches a new level of ridiculousness. Over the years I have had to amputate many tails either fully or partially through chronic, unhealing injury or trauma. Among the dogs these have been Staffies, a couple of Labradors, but most often greyhounds. Greyhounds are kennelled a lot of the time either in racing kennels or, unfortunately and all too commonly, in adoption centres once their racing days are over. Their tails are long and whip-like, and covered in particularly thin skin. Not a single pro-docker is suggesting they should be routinely docked. However, by far the highest number of tails I have amputated have been those of cats. They get run over, they get trapped in doors or underfoot, they get injured in fights and so on and so on. No one advocates the docking of cats' tails. Well, they use them for communication and balance, don't they? Hmm, sounds familiar …

My two wonderful dogs also had an 'enthusiastic tail action'. We developed amazing reflexes for grabbing glasses off the coffee table when one of them walked past it. They never hurt their tails. Should I have docked them on the off-chance or for my own convenience? I was walking my dogs one day and I saw a family coming towards me. I couldn't see any dogs at first and then three beautiful springers came tearing out of the bushes. Every one of them had a long, glorious tail and it made my day. They looked *so* happy. It was a joy to see. That got me thinking about the whole issue, as it does every time I see a docked dog or one that 'should' be but isn't.

If we extrapolate the injury argument to avoiding all injuries maybe we should do a trial. Let's see what would happen if we kept all dogs and cats indoors for a year. We would see no fight wounds, no cut pads, no grass seeds, no traffic accidents and virtually no lameness.

However, that situation has already happened to a lesser degree. During the foot-and-mouth outbreak of 2001 people couldn't exercise their dogs anywhere near as much as they would usually. The surgery in which I was working at the time was practically empty. Farm work was booming, but small animal work dropped off noticeably. My point was proved. It is *easy* to stop our dogs getting injured, but it wouldn't be acceptable to say we should just keep them indoors. Therefore it is just as unacceptable to dock dogs routinely just in case they injure their tail in later life.

There is one totally fundamental point to make here that was never said in any of the debates I have heard on this issue. The people who wish to continue docking to prevent tail injury and amputation are, in fact, injuring 100% of the animals concerned. With this in mind, if there was a total ban on all tail docking you would be improving the welfare of every single dog that *didn't* injure its tail later in life.

When the Animal Welfare Act was passed in Scotland they did the right thing and went for a complete ban across all breeds with no exemptions. In 2014 a study was done to try to assess the impact the ban had had on rates of tail injury. There were many people clamouring for a review and a possible introduction of exemptions. The study concluded that spaniels and hunt point retrievers had more injuries after the ban. Part of it was a little spurious because it was based on owners' recording of injuries, not vets. It found that around 17% of these breeds sustained an injury. Obviously they didn't all require treatment and certainly didn't all require amputation. However, even if every one of them had needed surgery the ban had effectively avoided amputation and improved welfare in **83%** of the dogs.

When the study looked at vet practice data it found that 0.53% of non-working breeds had tail injuries and 0.9% of working breeds did. The pro-dockers all started shouting from the rooftops about how working dogs are so much more prone to injury, *but* even in the working breeds, **99.1%** of them *didn't* injure their tails according to veterinary data. Avoiding injury does not stand up as an argument.

2. For Reasons of Hygiene

The CDB suggests that long-haired dogs such as Yorkies and Old English sheep-dogs should be docked because of the risk of faecal soiling, which could lead to fly strike and other serious health problems. We'll be looking at the outstanding hairiness of some of our dog breeds later, but surely if you have a dog whose coat is so untenable that it could get infested with maggots you need to either breed for shorter hair or keep the hair round its anus clean and clipped short. Cutting its tail off probably isn't going to make much difference if that's your level of monitoring!

Why are other long-haired breeds such as bearded collies and rough collies not docked? German shepherds are well known for being predisposed to a condition called anal furunculosis, which is a chronic, deep infection of the skin around the anus, in the worst cases leading to euthanasia. Why are they left with their tails? While we are on the subject, we may wonder why Persian cats aren't docked. All of this will soon become apparent when we look at reason three.

3. To Maintain Breed Standards

This is my personal favourite and is obviously the major, only thinly disguised, reason why tail docking has continued to happen. It is worth looking closely at the CDB argument here, so I will quote directly from its website:

> 'Breeds which have been docked over many generations have been selected for specific qualities of build and conformation, but not for tail length, shape or carriage. If left undocked, it is unlikely that the best dogs would carry good tails. In seeking to maintain the quality of the breeds, breeders would therefore be left with a diminished number of suitable sires and dams. The genetic pool would be reduced, greatly increasing the risk of hereditary diseases taking hold. Some breeds could even disappear forever.'

This honestly makes me laugh. I cannot believe that anyone would listen to such a load of tripe as this statement. How can a dog not have a 'good' tail? That is how they are born. The whole concept of the breed standard is an important cause of health problems and poor animal welfare in the UK and all over the world.

The above statement by the CDB actually says that breeders will be so concerned with how their show dog looks that they will ignore the gene pool because they are 'forced' to select for 'good tails'. If they actually cared about their animals they would select for healthy, whole dogs that can lead a normal life.

The RCVS guide to professional conduct has long stated that docking for breed type or conformation is unethical and the veterinary surgeon involved could be struck off the register for professional misconduct. It used terms such as 'conduct *disgraceful* in a professional respect' and '*unacceptable mutilation*' (my italics). Is the CDB honestly saying it knows more about the physiology and pain receptors of these dogs than the governing body of the veterinary profession?

Whenever I was presented with a docked puppy, usually for vaccination, I would mention it to the owners, though not in an accusatory way. I soon realised after talking to many owners that they simply had no idea about what went on or the reasons behind it. Most are horrified and will say they would have got a tailed one had they known. Prior to the partial ban I once met a new client under very sad circumstances. He is a loving owner and has had boxers for years. His very elderly boxer had had a massive fit and, although he recovered, after a few days of deterioration we decided the kindest thing to do was to put him to sleep. As I'm sure many of you can imagine, the man was heartbroken. A few days later he popped in to have a chat about things and bring in a thank you card. He had his young and very beautiful other dog with him. I thought that we knew each other well enough for me to broach the subject and I asked him about the docking situation. He asked about the procedure and the reasons and gave it some consideration. After a few seconds he said he would be more than happy to have a boxer with a tail because, spoken like what I would consider to be a true *lover* of the breed, he said, 'A boxer's a boxer to me whether it's got a tail or not. I'd definitely have one with a tail.' This heartened me greatly. Thankfully these days many breeds such as boxers that were traditionally docked in the UK are now commonly seen with wonderful tails.

The truth is that docking *is* painful. It takes away a dog's ability to communicate with other dogs, and there is the risk of haemorrhage at the time, spinal infections and even death. There is some evidence of a link between docking and problems with the nerve supply to the bladder and rectum; and between docking and the development of perineal hernias. I have seen puppies that chew their stump because of the discomfort. I have seen ones that knock the end of their stump every time they sit down. There is *no* excuse. I do actually have some experience in this respect because when I was 13 years old I had to have both my little toes amputated because of an issue when I was growing. I'd had two surgeries at 11 and 12 years of age to try to correct it, but then eventually the decision was made to lop them off. It's not unusual for me to knock the stumps of bone on passing

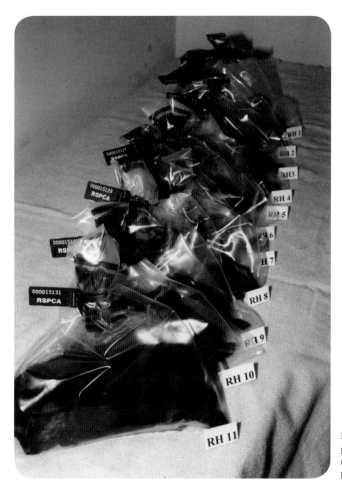

Figure 7.1: A litter of 11 puppies that died following tail docking with a Stanley knife. (Photo: RSPCA)

objects or when I exercise, and it hurts. I've seen many docked puppies sit down, but then keep standing up and trying again to sit comfortably. Many of these animals must experience this discomfort throughout their whole lives because of human vanity. It disgusts me.

In the Kennel Club book of 2004 there were around 50 breeds in which docking was optional or, in most cases, 'customary'. It also specified how much should be taken off to meet the breed standard. I have heard of judges that have held their hand up when judging to block the offending appendage from view. Indeed, the book tells you what the tail 'should' look like when it is present. In the case of the Old English sheepdog, which was customarily docked right to the base, the tail, when present, should be 'unobtrusive' and 'never curled or carried over back'. Was this so we could pretend it wasn't there? I once had the pleasure of seeing two undocked examples of this breed and the tail is like a wonderful, flag waving wildly in the breeze. No such thing should ever be made to be 'unobtrusive'. I'm very pleased to see that in the new standards of 2017 the tail should have, 'natural carriage'. Progress at last!

The fact is that I qualified in 1996 and I was not taught how to dock tails except therapeutically, just as with any surgical procedure. I don't know when the universities stopped teaching it, but it speaks volumes. I'm pretty sure that over time the practice will now just fizzle out simply because as younger vets come through there simply won't be anyone who will consider it ethical to perform it, whatever the law says about exemptions.

I'm over the moon that the law did change for many breeds. I was involved in several prosecutions after the law came into effect. Sadly, though we still see thousands of dogs docked under the exemptions, the vast majority of which will never be used for work. Even those that do work sometimes end up being gun shy and are rehomed as pets. Fundamentally, as the evidence shows, there is no need to dock working dogs either because the injury arguments simply don't stand up to scrutiny (see Figure 7.2 and 7.3).

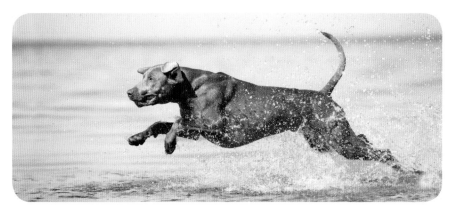

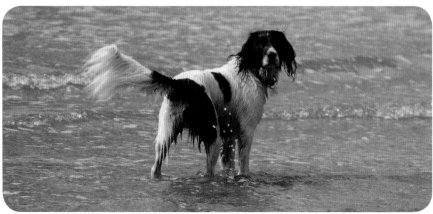

Figures 7.2, 7.3: Many owners happily work these dogs with wonderful full tails. (Photo: Adobe Stock)

I do feel as if times are changing and there are more and more beautiful tails wagging in this world than there were back then. I think we still have a long way to go with that though. If you are thinking of any breed of dog please make sure the breeder knows you'd like it whole!

In 2007 I wrote, at the end of this chapter, 'I hope that in 20 years' time children will look at old photos of docked dogs and wonder why on earth it went on in this day and age and be grateful that common sense prevailed.' Sadly that seems to be a long way off. To my horror and disappointment, in 2017, politicians in Scotland ignored a mountain of evidence and expert veterinary opinion, listened to the vocal interested parties once more and reversed their tail docking ban for certain working breeds. This is one of the biggest backward steps for animal welfare I've seen. In dog circles you will often hear the term 'fit for purpose'. We have to ask ourselves this; if working breeds are truly incapable of doing their work without risk of such serious injury that we need to pre-emptively amputate bits of their bodies are they fit for purpose? Apparently not. We have bred them to do a job for which they are not adequately robust so we either need to breed them to be stronger or stop expecting them to do that work. If we engage in 'sports' that require the mutilation of the animals involved then maybe we also need to ask some serious ethical questions about those 'sports'. As with my sentiment throughout this book, in the end, we should look back to nature and her examples. After all, wild canids hunt *really, really* well with their tails intact!

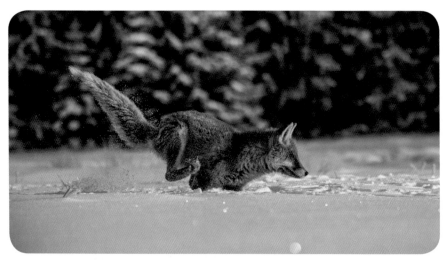

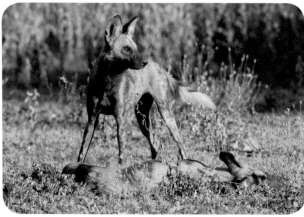

Figures 7.4, 7.5 : (Photo: Adobe Stock; Paul Joynson-Hicks)

Chapter 8

Hair – Too Much or Not Enough

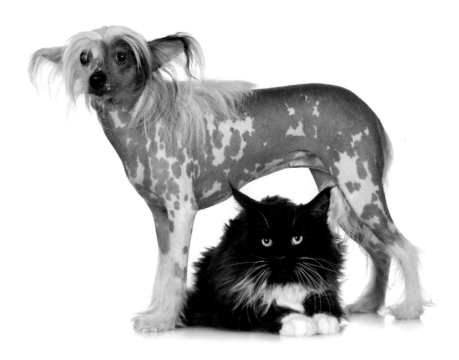

J UST THE SAME AS WITH THEIR BODIES, COATS ARE ONE OF THE THINGS WE have drastically changed in our dogs and cats without ever thinking about the consequences or the impact on them. I know it is wrong to assume dogs and cats have the same needs as us, but we are all mammals and I think we really need to start to empathise more. As this book is all about nature versus man I really think it's worth thinking about what evolution has selected for when it comes to hair. We need to consider how it changes between animal species, what its purpose is and how it differs on various body parts. Once we look at that it is so obvious to see where we have made such dreadful errors.

The wild canids and cats of varying sizes live in vastly different climates. From wolves and snow leopards in freezing parts to desert dwelling wild dogs and cats, the coats vary greatly, but they are not, ever, very long. Extremely long fur doesn't provide warmth, it hinders movement, makes you more likely to attract debris—either when trying to escape a predator or when you're hunting—makes you more

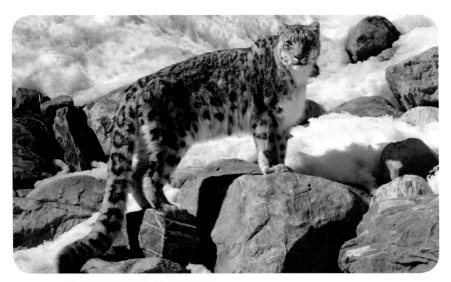

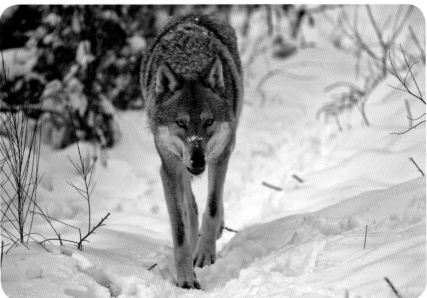

Figures 8.1, 8.2: Wild animals in cold climates have dense fur, not extremely long fur. (Photo: Adobe Stock)

prone to faecal soiling and fly strike and is impossible to keep clean, knot free or groom without human intervention. If you look at wild animals, even with their fullest winter coats in the harshest areas of the planet they rarely have extremely long fur and they never have long fur around their mouths.

Natural animals that need warmth from fur tend to have very dense coats and different types of layers to trap air and maintain warmth. They also rely on fat build-up over the summer to keep them warm through the winter. As the seasons change, or depending on the climate they live in, their coats change drastically throughout the year. I've often said to owners who are inundated with dog fur that if I could invent something to control or stop moulting I'd be a millionaire!

Of course, we don't expect our dogs and cats to live like wild animals in all sorts of conditions and catch their own food, but when you look at what excessive fur means for our animals we have still made life very difficult for some of them.

Let's talk about cats first. Cats are fastidious groomers, they hate being dirty and they love to climb and explore. Cats are also extremely sensitive creatures and find the smells of the perfumes and toiletries of the human world overpowering. It is very unnatural and often stressful for cats to be bathed, excessively handled and restrained, or even in some cases groomed. As soon as you give a cat a long coat you will change its life for the worse. Persians are the most notably affected. When you compare show-winning Persian cats from the early 1900s to those in the present they have changed beyond belief. Back then they had slightly shorter faces than a normal cat and slightly longer hair, more like a modern-day domestic long hair. In fact, Persians have become the very extreme modern types only since the 1960s and '70s. Now they have convex faces and the most unnatural, untenable hair imaginable. It's scary how quickly a breed can be deformed so drastically.

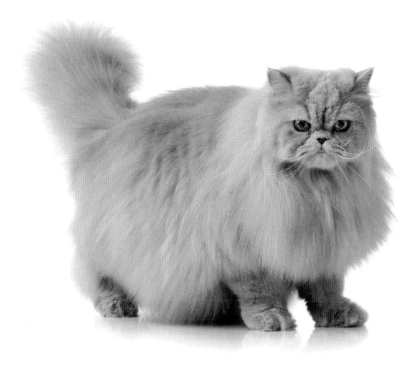

Figure 8.3: Very long coats can be extremely difficult to manage for owners and the cats themselves. (Photo: Adobe Stock)

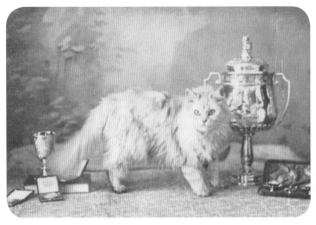

Figure 8.4: Persians at the turn of the century had coats like long-haired moggies. (Photo: Adobe Stock)

Some people with hours to spend on grooming do manage, but the cats need to be habituated from a very young age and it has to be consistent. Every small animal vet in the country will have de-matted a Persian cat. There are many owners who take them on without the slightest idea of the work they need to keep their coats free of knots; many are disheartened and frustrated. For us, it is also frustrating. Often the only solution is at best a sedative, at worst a full general anaesthetic, to sort them out. In many cases we have no option but to shave the whole cat apart from sometimes the head and tail. I've had cats brought in where literally the entire coat has come off in one solid mass like a sheep fleece. I can't imagine how

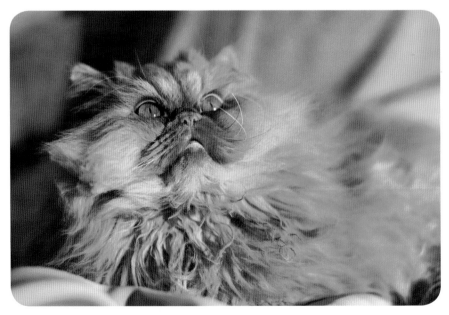

Figure 8.5: Imagine how matted fur must feel to a fastidious groomer. (Photo: Adobe Stock)

horrible this build-up of mats will be for a fastidious groomer like a cat. Add to that their abnormal faces and mouths and who knows what the life of a modern-day Persian might be like?

Having to sedate or anaesthetise animals for reasons brought about by cosmetic vanity is not why people become vets and it simply shouldn't happen. Any cats with long fur can have issues, so please think very carefully before taking one on or avoid them altogether. I know there will be people who disagree with me and say that with the correct grooming and bathing these cats are fine, but having to bath cats is totally absurd and perpetuating animals that need this level of maintenance for anything approaching a normal life is unacceptable.

And now let us turn our attention to dogs. To start with the most basic thing, long fur, as we said, is not natural; it hinders your movement and is difficult to keep clean. If you are low to the ground, or have hair that reaches to or almost to the ground, you will be hindered and you will gather all sorts of twigs and grass seeds when you go for a walk.

As I said, wild canids do not have long fur round their mouth. We have created many dog breeds in which a beard is considered desirable; I say desirable because it's the sort of language humans use and it is only us that desire them in dogs.

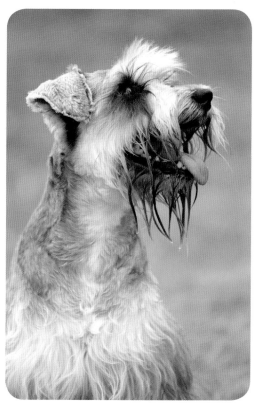

Figure 8.6: A soggy beard constantly dragged into your mouth can't be pleasant. (Photo: Adobe Stock)

Dogs' beards trap food and saliva, and often either smell, and are soggy with such trappings, or require another unnatural daily regime to keep them as clean as possible. You will often see the very clear saliva staining in the beards of the lighter-coloured dogs. Some dogs with long hair around their mouths also get hair caught and entwined in their teeth, which gets dragged in when they lick their lips. This can lead to infected gums and a great deal of discomfort.

One of my most resounding memories from being in practice was one such case. I finished writing up the notes from the patient I had just seen and opened the consulting room door to call in my next patient. The practice that I worked in at the time had about a 5m passage between the consult room and the waiting room. Even from where I was standing in my doorway I was hit by the most overpoweringly disgusting smell.

A couple walked in with their standard poodle and with them the stench became intensely worse. Many vets are used to pretty rank smells and it comes with the job, but this was on a whole different level. When I asked what the problem was they, astoundingly, announced that they, '… had recently started to notice a *little bit of a smell* when the dog *kissed* them.'

I don't know if I managed to hide the surprise on my face that they had not been overcome by the smell of pus from being in the same room as the dog, let alone the idea of letting it approach your face!

I agreed that he was indeed a little bit on the whiffy side and dared to open his mouth. The dog had months' worth of long matted fur entwined around all his bottom teeth. The hair had gradually become packed further and further down into his gum pockets around his teeth and had subsequently become infected. By the time I saw him his whole mouth was a pus-filled, rotting mess, with many of his teeth only being held in by the festering fur.

After extensive dental work and some much-needed antibiotics, the owners and, more importantly, the dog were very much happier.

Some breeds of dog with very long fur, such as Old English sheepdogs, are traditionally clipped in the summer, but then there are many breeds with equally long fur that are not. I've encountered owners of both Shelties and bearded collies that have looked horrified at the idea of clipping them in case, 'their coat didn't come back the same' or 'they wouldn't look like beardies anymore'.

I'm always tempted to suggest to those owners that in that case they should wear all their winter clothes all through the summer and see if they feel comfortable. Dogs don't sweat through their skin the way we do. They have some sweat glands on the pads of their feet, but they rely on panting for the majority of their cooling requirements. If we don't take off some of their 'clothes' it is exactly the same as us being denied the ability to cool down, so why won't some owners empathise?

I also think it's very important to consider coat types and breeds depending on where you live, too. Some breeds of dog have been categorically bred to have thick, warm coats for the jobs for which they were intended; huskies and the other sled dogs are the obvious example. If you live in the south of France, having a dog bred for the Arctic probably isn't going to be very fair on the poor creature.

Even besides the breeds that are traditionally clipped, there are many that aren't and this doesn't mean they *can't* be. Breeds such as collies, retrievers and shepherds could benefit massively from being clipped in the summer.

My dogs Pan and Badger were collie crosses. They were quite different and the whole litter was an accidental mating between a farm collie bitch and an unknown mongrel. The result was 13 wonderful and individual crosses. Badger had pretty normal fur, but Pan had very thick, woolly under-fur like a wolf.

One day, when Pan was about three years old, I noticed how he seemed to be struggling in the heat on one of our favourite summer walks. Badger was tearing around like his usual self, but Pan was plodding along next to me.

I took him to the surgery after our walk and set about him with a pair of clippers. Now, I am no groomer, had no clipper guards at the time and to be frank I made an awful job of it. At one point Pan looked round at himself, sighed deeply and adopted an Eeyore pose of deep resignation. By the time I had finished he was surrounded by enough fur to make two more dogs and had completely changed colour because his undercoat is very light grey as opposed to his usual black. The general consensus among the others at work was that Pan would be the laughing stock of his doggy friends. Regardless of all this, I took him back to our favourite hill that same afternoon and he ran about like a puppy. He was literally a different dog. After that he was clipped every summer as often as he needed doing and it categorically improved his life and his enjoyment of walks.

I met a very nice man at the beach once who was the proud owner of a clipped Border collie. We got talking, as dog owners often do. We were extolling the virtues of the clipped dog, not least because of the reduction in fur to be vacuumed up at home. He commented that when he had told his sister that he intended to clip the dog she had told him he simply couldn't because collies aren't normally clipped. This is a really common scenario. Why should it matter if they are usually clipped or not? When I go out on a hot day I don't wear all my winter clothes, so why do we expect our dogs to do the same?

A very dear and long-standing client of mine used to have a Sheltie called Duke. Duke developed heart failure as he got older and started struggling with his respiration. He responded well to medication, but obviously there is only so much the drugs can do. I saw him one day in the summer and Duke was heaving and panting. I suggested to Chris that he take Duke to the groomers and have him

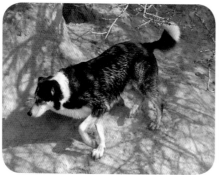
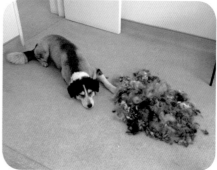
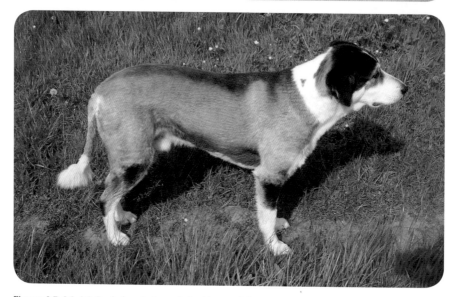

Figures 8.7, 8.8, 8.9: Pan before, during and after his annual clip!

clipped. I also told him to make sure they really 'buzzed' him. I saw them both the following week for a check-up and couldn't help laughing, as I had done with Pan. He looked totally different and we both had a chuckle over the new, slimline Duke. Anyway, it helped him enormously and took one more strain off his heart.

My husband, who is also a vet, also often suggests clipping to his clients since seeing the difference it made to Pan. He once had a client in with two Shelties and he had suggested having them clipped. The owner declined on the grounds that 'it would take all year to grow back'. Who cares? The point is that your dog really has no concept of how bad its haircut is or how different it looks. It will, however, experience the enormous relief that we get when we peel off layers of clothes when we are sweating like a pig.

When we do clip dogs there are many breeds that have it dictated which bits should be clipped. How many dogs do you see such as the schnauzer and the Cesky

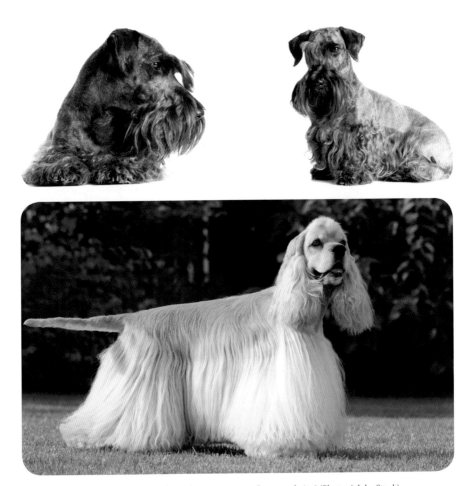

Figures 8.10, 8.11, 8.12: Why do we leave the most unnatural areas so hairy? (Photo: Adobe Stock)

terrier that have their bodies clipped, but the most annoying fur over their eyes and round their mouth left long? The cocker spaniel and Westies, to name just a couple, have a hovercraft-style skirt left behind that must be a nightmare on walks.

The ornamental clipping of poodles leaves me speechless. Indeed, the Kennel Club book of 2004 states that, 'for the fashion-conscious there are many different styles in which he can be clipped. A dandy at heart, he will always show his appreciation when his toilette has been completed.' I suspect dogs 'showing their appreciation' are just relieved to be off the groomer's table and allowed to be free again.

Flicking through the breed standards, there are dozens of dogs shown with different types of unnatural coats that for many owners will be hard work or will need regular trips to the groomer. We have even made breeds with dreadlocks such as the Komondor, Hungarian puli and Bergamasco. The breed description for all

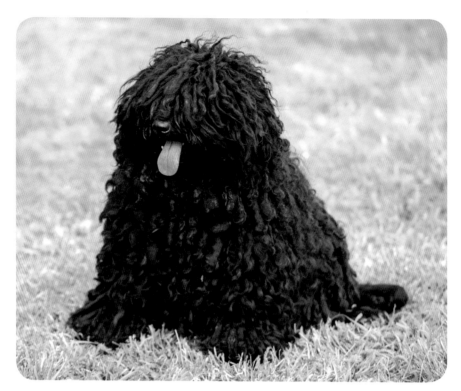

Figure 8.13: This simply can't be comfortable. (Photo: Adobe Stock)

of them states the coat naturally cords or mats to provide insulation in areas such as the Alps and keeps them fit for function. I question this. The pictures all show matted fur down to the ground and obscured eyes and vision. Having seen snow pack on to the foot fur of even normally coated dogs, I find it hard to imagine that floor-length, matted hair in the snow and not being able to see really aids your herding ability. I'm not a shepherd though, so I may well be wrong!

There are more than 30 breeds shown in the breed standard book, including the Yorkie, Skye terrier, otterhound, Irish water spaniel, Spanish water dog, Cesky terrier, Scottish terrier, Sealyham terrier, Skye terrier, wheaten terrier, Lhasa apso, poodles, schnauzer, shih-tzu, Tibetan terrier, Bouvier, Portuguese water dog, Russian black terrier, bearded collie, Bergamasco, Briard, Catalan sheepdog, puli, Komondor, OESD, Polish lowland sheepdog, Bolognese, Chinese crested, Coton de Tulear, Havanese, Lowchen, and the Maltese, that all have their vision obscured by their hair. Sorry to list so many, but we need to see the extent of what we have done. Let's not forget the Pekingese. This breed has the most outrageously unnatural coat you can imagine combined with extreme brachycephaly.

Some people will, of course, clip the fur away from the eyes or use hair bands to hold it back, but many won't. How many humans would choose to constantly obscure their vision? Maybe some of the teenage fashions where I suspect it's more about annoying their parents than a desire to not be able to see very well. How many wild canids and cats have their vision obscured or long hair around their mouths? None. Zero.

One of the consequences that even fewer people consider with all these aberrations is the effect it has on the ability of our dogs to communicate with each other. Dogs display a large number of signals that express their mood and how they feel when encountering any other dog. A confident dog will stand very erect, prick up its ears and hold its tail erect. A less confident dog will flatten its ears, may cower and have its tail down or at 'half-mast'. A threatened dog may raise its hackles. Eye contact, or lack of it, is also very important.

Dogs that have very long, heavy ears cannot prick their ears, very shaggy dogs cannot raise their hackles and dogs without tails can do very little to communicate at all. I was once talking to a very good behavioural specialist and I asked him if he encountered many behavioural problems in docked dogs. He said that, yes, he did see some, but the worst for him was the Old English sheepdog. I had never really considered this before, but could immediately see what he meant. These dogs' faces, lips and ears are covered in hair, they cannot effectively raise their hackles, they cannot make or avoid eye contact and 99% of them used to be docked (and still are in some countries). We have effectively made these dogs mute. Dogs that cannot communicate can have problems in that they can sometimes draw aggression because other dogs are unsure about how to approach when they meet.

Of course, humans, in their role of the thorn in Mother Nature's side, have also gone to the other extreme and deemed it a good idea to produce animals with little or no fur at all. The Sphynx cat and Chinese crested dog spring straight to mind. The

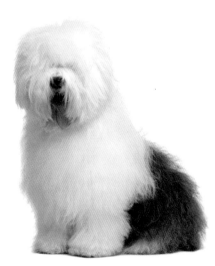

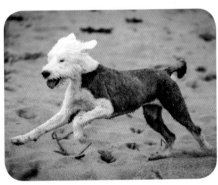

Figures 8.14, 8.15: Which dog can express themselves more clearly? (Photo: Adobe Stock)

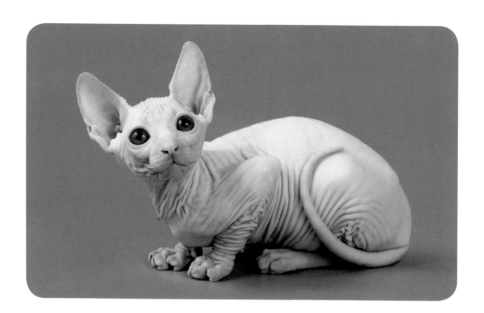

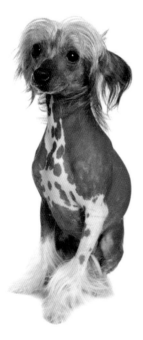

Figures 8.16, 8.17: Hairless animals have multiple issues to contend with and are unprotected from sunburn and injury. (Photo: Adobe Stock)

genetics of hairlessness varies between breeds, but in these two breeds if a puppy or kitten gets two copies of the gene they die in the womb and will not develop.

When Sphynx cats first started to be bred there were many stories of either lack of conception, poor libido or kittens dying that the breed has ended up only being maintained through outcrossing to breeds such as the rex. For the Chinese crested dogs you will get some puppies with hair and some without, and some combinations in between that often apparently end up being shaved to conform to the hairless breed standard.

All hairless dogs and cats are at risk of sunburn and skin cancer, heat loss and hypothermia in cold climates and they require bathing and some care to keep the build-up of oil off their skin, which hair would naturally absorb and distribute. They are, of course, also prone to injury because they are unprotected by fur. Sphynx cats can have ear problems because their lack of fur means that more dirt and debris ends up in the ear rather than being trapped in the guard hairs of normal animals. They also have mutated or absent whiskers, another part of a 'whole, natural cat' that is very important to daily sensations. The brilliant charity and cat welfare organisation International Cat Care is as succinct and to the point as we all should be when it says of the sphynx, 'For a cat, a coat is essential. We should not be breeding hairless cats.'

Many people cite these animals as being less allergenic for owners, but this is not true. Most human allergies are to dander or skin proteins and saliva rather than to fur, so in fact sometimes allergies are worse in the presence of a hairless animal.

Many owners of hairless cats have to keep them indoors to avoid fight wounds, other injuries and sun damage. Being kept solely indoors is a huge cause of stress and frustration for many cats. Hairless dogs and cats can often be seen wearing jumpers and coats. Doesn't anyone think it might be better to leave them with the coats that nature gave them?

All these coat and hair aberrations are more examples of how we have become so obsessed with what our animals look like that we have forgotten to consider the impact on them. Your dog or cat has no concept of looks or beauty. Breed differences are a totally fabricated, man-made phenomenon. We need to start thinking about the day-to-day needs of our animals, not whether they conform to a popular idea of what a certain dog or cat 'should' look like.

Chapter 9

Teacups and Giants

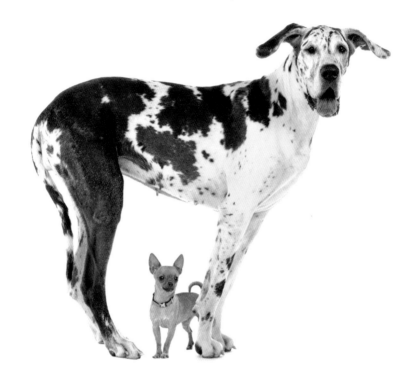

O NE OF THE BIGGEST DRIVERS OF POPULARITY WITH CERTAIN BREEDS is celebrity owners. You have your greats such as Paul O'Grady, Tom Hardy and Ricky Gervais who strongly support adoption and cross-breeds, but then there are many who love quirky breeds and flaunt them publicly seemingly to attention seek. In these days of social media there are freakish dogs and cats that become internet sensations because they are so 'hilariously' ugly or weird. It's really horrible.

Small dogs have become more and more popular, driven hugely by some very notable celebrities parading around with dogs in handbags and also by social media trending. Of course, some people have opted for small dogs because of where they live or their lifestyle. The problem is that producing increasingly unnaturally small and fragile dogs to suit a whim or a lifestyle choice of ours is still detrimental to the animals.

I have always been a firm believer that having animals is a privilege, not a right. Just because you want a dog or cat, or any animal for that matter, does not mean you should have it. If you don't have time to exercise a dog or you live in a flat, which means a cat can't have freedom, then maybe you have to put the animals' needs before your own and either choose a different pet or realise you may need to wait until your circumstances change.

For hundreds of years we've had smaller dogs and bigger dogs, but with all these breeding quirks we have gone way too far. We now see many small breeds becoming progressively smaller or with deteriorating health. As we said with the bowed legs in the earlier chapters, many small breed dogs have issues with their joints, both through shape of the legs and also with things such as luxating knee caps or patellae, but for some 'toy' breeds the problems are much more serious.

I think it's worth taking a second or two to reflect on the fact that we even have a division of dogs called toys. The Kennel Club breed standard book tells us that in days gone by Pekes were carried in the sleeves of kimonos and in Europe little dogs were carried around in baskets and were the 'toys' of the ladies of the household. It tells us that many toy breeds were miniature versions of sporting equivalents and suggests that the breeds may have started because the runts of sporting dogs were given to ladies who bred them for their 'diminutive size, charm and personality'.

Of course, over time we have had many traditions in animal keeping that we have realised are inappropriate and outdated now we have a better understanding of animal health and welfare. Perhaps it's worth wondering if creating entire breeds out of the puppies that were least likely to survive was probably not the best idea.

Toy breeds such as the Chihuahua, Maltese terrier and Yorkshire terrier have a higher than normal incidence of hydrocephalus, commonly called water on the brain. This condition is where fluid builds up and it can cause pressure on the brain, nervous signs, pain, nausea and also thinning and doming of the bones of the skull. It's a difficult condition to treat and can cause lifelong suffering and often early euthanasia. No one understands exactly why these animals are more likely to suffer, but it seems likely that, as with the soft tissue in the mouths of the brachys, changing the size of one part of the dog does not necessarily change the rest. By making the skulls of these small breeds so small we have somehow changed the relationship with the size of the brain.

The most shocking example of this is the case of chiari-like malformation and syringomyelia (CM/SM) in Cavalier King Charles spaniels (CKCS). This condition was a major feature of the *Pedigree Dogs Exposed* programme of 2008 and caused a huge outcry from the public at the suffering of these animals. Cavaliers have somehow become a special case when it comes to skull and brain mismatching. It's not fully understood, but is probably because of the smaller skull and also its shape that has been selected over time in these dogs. Their brain size has remained that of a bigger dog and their skull has become not only smaller but domed or boxy, which has made the mismatch more pronounced. Studies are widely ongoing into this disease, but it was first diagnosed in 1997 and the prevalence seems to be rising. Studies suggest that up to 75% of CKCS may be affected by at least one abnormality and probably around 5% are clinically affected. You may think this is a small number, but it equates to thousands of dogs worldwide and is something that breeders should be absolutely prioritising to try to breed it out.

CM/SM, in its most basic description, is a brain that bulges out of the back of the skull because it has nowhere else to go. The pressure created at the base of the skull causes fluid to build up in the spinal cord and brain. I'm sure you can imagine that something as important as your brain hanging out into your spinal cord is never going to be something you would hope for. There is a whole spectrum of severity in these dogs and some can live a pain-free life and seem largely unaffected. The mild cases often present to vets as dogs with ear problems or even fleas because they scratch at their ears and the backs of their necks. The most severe cases scream in pain and writhe on the floor, and are incredibly distressing (see Figure 9.1–9.4).

Drugs can sometimes help and surgery is possible for some cases, but many of the more severe ones end up being euthanased because of the uncontrollable pain. Specialist neurologists helped set up a screening scheme for CM/SM to try to reduce the incidence, but the scheme has sadly, to date, been largely ignored by breeders. We'll be talking about health testing in much more detail in the following

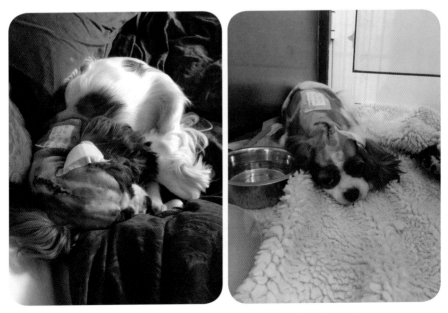

Figures 9.1, 9.2: Some dogs' suffering can be alleviated with neurosurgery. (Photo: Emma Bennett)

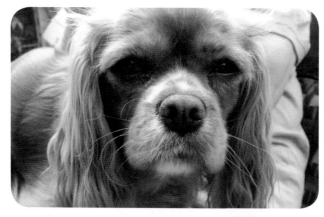

Figure 9.3: Many Cavaliers have chronic headaches and suffer in silence. (Photo: Sheila Nolan)

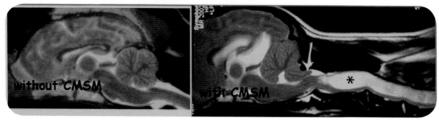

Figure 9.4: MRI shows the normal brain on the left. On the right the arrow shows where the brain bulges out of the back of the skull. You can see large white areas in the middle of the brain where fluid has built up. The large fluid-filled syrinx shown by the asterisk in the spinal cord compresses the cord, but also damages the areas above and below it as well. (Photo: Clare Rusbridge and Penny Knowler)

chapters, but for now it's important to remember that even clinically unaffected dogs, if not screened, will be passing on the abnormalities to some offspring that could be more likely to develop the disease.

So toy and small dogs have their issues, but in recent years we've seen the exaggeration to the teacup dogs; people apparently striving to try and create dogs that are as small as possible. As with our ancestors, it seems now that people are taking the runts of the original runts and breeding for increasingly small size. Runts are often small because of congenital problems and using them to breed is simply idiotic.

Teacup dogs are prone to heart disease, hypoglycaemia (low blood sugar), tracheal collapse, knee problems, weak bones, liver shunts, seizures, respiratory problems and blindness. Because of their size, they are less likely to cope with the cold and also much more likely to be seriously hurt or killed by accidental injuries. If you like animals the size of rats or guinea pigs maybe you should consider rats or guinea pigs instead of dogs. They too have welfare needs, so do your research, but taking one species and changing it to suit our desires is unacceptable and fraught with problems.

Do *not* buy or breed teacup dogs please.

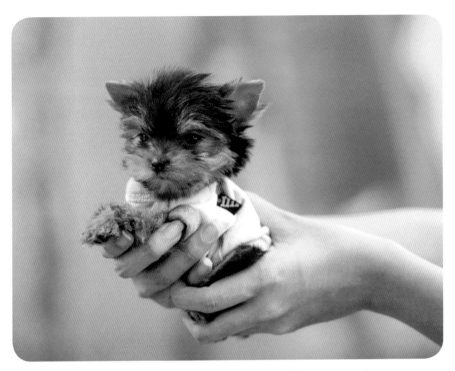

Figure 9.5: Dogs that are too fragile to go on the floor are not really dogs! (Photo: Adobe Stock)

On the opposite end of the spectrum are the giants. Most people are aware of the phrase, 'the bigger they are, the harder they fall', but when it comes to our dog breeds the end of the saying should be, '... the younger they die.'

Giant breeds are dogs such as the St Bernard, Newfoundland, mastiffs, Irish wolfhound, Leonberger and, of course, the epitome of the giants, the Great Dane. When I was in practice I heard many people say of such dogs, 'They're too big for their hearts.' The truth is that these giant breeds and other larger breeds have an array of health problems, just one of which is a shocking level of heart disease and premature death.

An article in the *Veterinary Record* in 1999 by A.R. Michell looked at the 'longevity of British breeds of dog and its relationships with sex, size, cardiovascular variables and disease'. Of the dogs in the study it found that the Bernese mountain dog, bull mastiff, flat-coated retriever, Great Dane, Irish wolfhound, Rhodesian ridgeback, Rottweiler and the St Bernard all had median ages at death of less than nine years. By contrast, Jack Russells, toy poodles, whippets, some terriers and, of course, the good old cross-breed had median ages of more than 13 years, almost 50% longer than their large counterparts. This would be like one family of humans dying on average 30 years earlier than others. You'd soon start to question why and try to avoid these young deaths.

The fact is that with so many of these cases we have come to accept it as the norm. I know many people who would not be at all surprised if their giant dog died at the age of eight. Indeed, they are often surprised if they last any longer. The fact is that we *should* be questioning this. Of course we should. We live in an age where the advances in veterinary medicine and surgery are akin to human medicine. Life expectancy should be going up across the board for humans and animals alike. For moggie cats and many true cross-breed dogs this is the case. When I was a child the average life expectancy of dogs was about 12 and cats about 13. These days many dogs live to 15 or 16 and it's certainly not uncommon to have cats of 18-20 years of age. So why are large and giant dogs, and some of the smaller pedigree breeds for that matter, dying so young?

I would have been horrified if any of my cross-breeds had died much earlier than they did, let alone *seven or eight years* before they did. It is the same as people accepting that bulldogs snore. This is not normal and it should not be considered normal any more.

When I worked in Tewkesbury I had the great pleasure to meet a young woman named Rachel and her first ever dog, Dudley. He was a gorgeous eight-week-old Great Dane. She absolutely adored him. Because he was a Dane we carefully went into all the reasons why she had to be careful with his nutrition and speed of growth. These breeds are predisposed to growth problems and joint problems because of the sheer extent of growing they have to do. They should be matured relatively slowly so that everything has time to develop properly, a bit like a good wine!

He had a few normal puppy problems but nothing major. We had him in regularly because we were tracking his growth carefully. We all became very attached to him. Just after he turned one, Rachel went on a well-deserved holiday. Dudley was left in the hands of some very good friends with a large house and a large garden.

I was driving home for a rare lunch break one day when I had a call from the surgery asking me to go on an urgent visit to these people's house where they 'thought Dudley was dead'. This seemed incredible to me and I thought there must be some misunderstanding or crossed wires somewhere along the line. I drove straight to the house and there he was, flat out on one side in the garden, stone dead. It was a beautiful sunny day and the carers had been pottering about in the garden and Dudley was loping around intermittently chasing butterflies and sleeping in the shade of a big tree. One minute he had been fine and the next dead. I was devastated and I knew that Rachel would be absolutely distraught because she had devoted so much to him. He was such a sweet dog too; it just seemed unbelievable. He had died of an acute heart problem. For him it was probably a blessing. He was playing in the sun and then there was nothing. Many of these dogs develop heart disease and can endure a prolonged decline, usually requiring months, if not years of medication. At least he was spared that.

The truth is that I have seen at least two other Danes die of heart failure before the age of four, even though I don't see many Danes. I know we love these gentle giants, but isn't it time we let them shrink a little? I met a man in the village we used to live in near York out walking once with what I learned was his third Dane. We got talking and he informed me proudly that all his had lasted until they were ten to 12 years old. This is sadly becoming rarer and rarer. He then went on to say that they always picked the smallest dog in the litter. This worked well for him and his dogs. Having said that, I also know that one of Mark's clients who dotes on his Dane also got the smallest one and she has had a lifetime at the surgery for one thing or another.

The most common heart disease they are affected by is dilated cardiomyopathy (DCM). This is basically a disease in which the heart gets progressively larger and the walls of the pumping chambers, the ventricles, become thinner and weaker. With time the heart becomes like a floppy water-balloon and its pumping power is seriously reduced, with heart failure and death being an inevitable end point.

One study found that 35.5% of Great Danes are affected with DCM. The breeds most likely to suffer are the likes of St Bernards and Newfoundlands. Dobermanns are reported to have a prevalence of a whopping 45–63%. Irish wolfhounds are 38 times more likely to have DCM than mixed breeds, and the Neapolitan mastiff is 40 times more likely to have it. These are shocking numbers.

Besides heart disease, there are also other conditions that are much more likely to be seen in giant breeds or the larger or heavier breeds, such as Rottweilers, setters, Labradors and retrievers, and hounds, such as the bloodhound. The growth diseases we see such as hip dysplasia, elbow dysplasia and OCD are more commonly seen among these dogs. Many of these breeds are also unfortunately predisposed to bone tumours and other cancers. Many bone tumours are incredibly aggressive, very painful and have very poor survival rates (see Figure 9.6).

I once had a client with a beautiful Rottie called Alice. She was an absolutely wonderful patient and had a great temperament. She had come in at the age of seven with lameness. She was a very big dog and we hoped she had just overdone it. However, with the breed diagnostic tool we use so often she had a different list of differentials to a mongrel or, for that matter, most small dogs. She showed very little response to pain relief and a swelling appeared rapidly over the following few days. X-rays and further tests confirmed our worst fears that a tumour was present and Alice had to be euthanased within weeks because of the pain. It was a tragic case, as was the skull tumour I saw in 2005 in another very sweet Rottie called Petra. These animals and their owners went through horrible times that may not have happened before breeding went too far.

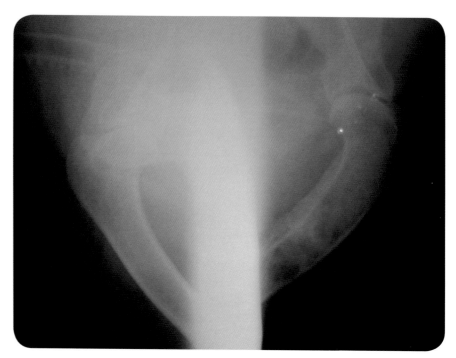

Figure 9.6: Bone tumour on the right compared to normal bone on the left.

The Kennel Club undertook surveys in 2004 and 2014 to assess pedigree dog health. The individual results for each breed and for each year can be found on its website and make interesting reading. The overall life expectancy of *all* dogs has gone from 11 to ten years between the two surveys, i.e. it has got worse. The KC does take pains to point out that the two surveys were very different, so should not be directly compared. It will be interesting to see if a 2024 survey matches the sampling techniques for 2014 so that we *can* actually compare the data.

According to the 2014 survey, the giant breeds are indeed dying very young and often of bone tumours, other cancers and heart disease. A quarter of Irish wolfhounds died of heart disease and 12.5% of bone tumours. Their median life span was a paltry six and a half years, about the same as a guinea pig. Great Danes live a little longer with a median of seven years, but almost a third of them die of heart failure. For Rottweilers the cancer statistics are shocking, with almost 45% of them dying of some kind of tumour, but the trophy for the breed most blighted by cancer goes to the poor flat-coated retriever with a staggering **56%** dying of some form of cancer. These life expectancies and levels of disease are certainly nothing of which breed clubs should be proud (see Figure 9.7).

The giant breeds are also candidates for one of the most life-threatening emergencies as well – bloat. Gastric dilatation and volvulus (GDV), as it's properly

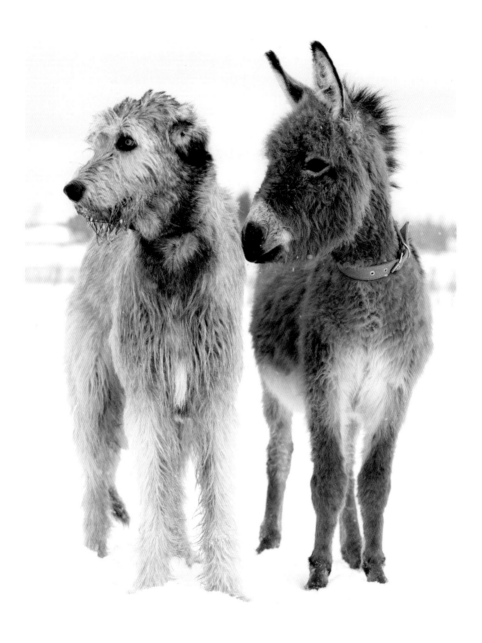

Figure 9.7: Sadly, dogs as big as donkeys aren't destined for long lives. (Photo: Adobe Stock)

named, is still a bit of a mystery. It's thought that it may be related to the very deep chest of some dogs, but this has never been proven. Certainly when you look at the breeds most commonly affected—setters, Great Danes, wolfhounds, mastiffs and Newfoundlands—they do certainly all seem to have that in common.

For some reason, usually after eating, these dogs sometimes get an incredibly swollen stomach full of gas and literally expand in front of your eyes. They often look like they are trying to be sick, but nothing comes out. If you see this go straight to your vet without hesitation. Only about 50% of these dogs survive. In many the stomach twists (the volvulus in GDV) on itself and this can lead to shock, septicaemia and death within hours if not treated.

We must remember too that cats are starting to be tinkered with and exaggerated in the same way as dogs. Many owners of large and giant dogs and cats love to tell people how big they are and how much they weigh. It's like a badge of honour to have the biggest of something. It somehow reflects some of that glory that means nothing at all to the animal back on to the owner. In cats the giants are the Maine Coons. They too are not uncommonly affected by heart disease and joint problems, most commonly hip dysplasia. Hip dysplasia is very common in certain breeds of dog, but virtually unheard of in moggie cats and can cause cripplingly painful arthritis. For great explorers and climbers such as cats its effect on quality of life can be devastating, as of course it can be for dogs.

As with all things in life, moderation is the key. If you don't want a medium-sized dog or cat think long and hard about the opposite ends of the size spectrum. Think about the impact that choice could have on your bank account, your emotions and, most importantly, the breed of animal you will be perpetuating demand for that could continue to be plagued by breed-related disease and early death.

Chapter 10

Inherited Disease – One Day Son, All This Could Be Yours!

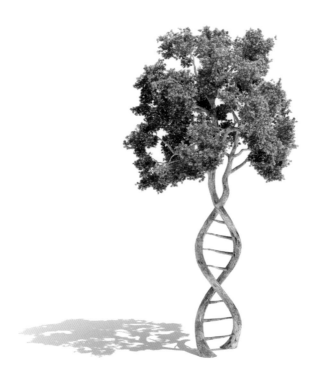

ONE OF THE THINGS I ABSOLUTELY LOVE ABOUT MY JOB IS THE CLIENTS; they are a constant surprise and it is one of the things that makes the job interesting. In small-animal work we often see people for very short, intense periods of time, so it is difficult to get to know them unless you see them very frequently or work somewhere for a long time. Once I had a client who came in with his Scottish deerhound. I'd seen him a few times previously for boosters for this dog and their lurcher. This time the deerhound had a very swollen and painful eye and I had asked him to come back to see me to make sure the problem was totally sorted. The client is a doctor who works in accident and emergency and has always been lovely to deal with. (I suspect doctors and vets encounter a lot of the same frustrations!)

On the day of the check-up I was very pleased to see that the eye was fully returned to normal and his owner was just about to leave when he said, 'You know, I'm sure these things are getting overbred. Just look how deep his eyes are in the sockets.' I said that I was glad he had opened up about it and told him about my concerns with our pedigrees. He said (and this is what I mean when I say clients are a constant, refreshing surprise), 'I know. When we got him we were given this 15-generation pedigree and it's all the same [expletive deleted] names on it!' Well, I had to chuckle. It's rare that people are that open about something and I was pleased he felt he could be with me.

The point of the story is that he was absolutely right to not only notice this fact, but also recognise it as a problem. As I said before, in practice I was often presented with a new puppy or kitten and the proud owner would produce the pedigree certificate with a theatrical flourish and show it to me. Some would tell me that they had even paid extra for the longer ones with more generations on it. The same names used to crop up time and again where closely related animals had been bred together. Line breeding, as it's called, is what we would generally call incest if it were a human family. It's still very popular (line breeding that is, not incest!), with some breeders of the opinion that it is the only way to ensure the 'purest of pedigrees'.

The UK Kennel Club has finally outlawed close line breeding and states that puppies will not be registered if, 'The offspring are the result of any mating between father and daughter, mother and son or brother and sister, save in exceptional circumstances or for scientifically proven welfare reasons.' The GCCF also warns against these matings for cats, using the words 'full siblings'. Does this mean that you could have two litters from the same pair at different times and mate the offspring together? I don't know. You'll notice that it is still considered acceptable in dogs and cats to mate grandparents with grandsons and granddaughters, and presumably aunts, uncles and cousins are all fair game. It all still feels a bit unsavoury to me.

That beautiful, strong woman, Mother Nature, has ways of dealing with line breeding in the wild. Firstly, some animals naturally disperse or kick their young out at a certain age. This means the offspring wander off and find other groups, which keeps the gene pool fresh and diverse. Those that do stay in close groups will sometimes welcome newcomers, adding new genetic material, but also, and fundamentally, any close mating that produces an unhealthy individual results in disease and death, thereby stopping those genes being continued, always selecting for health. Which is, of course, the key to survival of the fittest!

According to the *Collins English Dictionary*, the history of the word 'pedigree' comes from the Old French *pie de grue*, 'crane's foot', alluding to the spreading lines used in a genealogical chart. In simple terms, it just means a family tree.

Knowing this, I have pondered why the word conjures up the notion of a higher class of animal. Why do we feel that pedigrees are more desirable than a cross-breed?

I think there are several reasons. Firstly, we pay a large amount of money for them. This appeals to our subconscious perception of worth. Surely a £1000 pedigree is 'better' than a £100 mongrel dog from the local adoption centre in the same way that a £100,000 sports car is 'better' than a £10,000 hatchback. Extending this analogy it's the same with the insurance. Pedigrees are often more expensive to insure than cross-breeds. Some owners seem to view this as a sign of the worth or prowess of their pure bred animal. In fact it is simply that they are more likely to end up needing veterinary treatment than a good old healthy cross-breed, just the same as that sports car that costs the same as a small house will have *very* expensive parts.

Secondly, I think it is because the word 'pedigree' is often used interchangeably with the word 'purebred'. The word pure also conjures up images of untainted and unspoilt lineage. Thirdly, I believe it is marketing over the years from companies that use the word pedigree, such as Pedigree pet foods and Pedigree ales. We always associate the word with the best of the best, but this is far from true when it comes to our dogs and cats. If a pedigree is a family tree then many these days are covered in mouldy fruit.

Most of what I have told you so far are problems that our dogs and cats have because of the shapes we have imposed on them. I wanted to make the problems appear separate from inherited disease because I really want you to start considering the deviations in shape from the starting point of the wild cats and canids and because I think looking at body shape makes these deformities easier to see and understand. However, by the very nature of the fact that it is the physical characteristics that have dictated the selection of these animals the problems associated with body shape are also inherited. In this chapter I want to examine the other diseases and conditions that have been inadvertently and unwittingly selected for alongside the outward appearance of the animals.

The sad fact is that there are now over *seven hundred* inherited or predisposed conditions in our pedigree dog and cat breeds. By predisposed I mean that we see a higher incidence of some conditions in certain breeds, even though the exact mode of inheritance has yet to be found. Nonetheless they are well documented and well recognised by vets. As I said, this doesn't happen in nature. *Breeds* would simply not exist. Over the hundred or so years that man has really got fervent about breeding and making these animals so 'pure' we have reduced gene pools to stagnant, filthy puddles in some cases. This unprecedented level of disease can only continue because of the advances in veterinary medicine and surgery. It is way past time we see the unacceptable nature of what we've done and do something positive to make amends.

The list of inherited problems is, as you may well imagine, very long and very complex. What stuns me is that we have got to this point. The veterinary profession knows all about it, the Kennel Club and Cat Fancy associations know all about it, but the public are still being led to believe that by buying a pedigree dog or cat they are buying the best animal they can get. With the recent booming popularity of the most deformed of pedigrees, the brachycephalics, it would seem we really have hit rock bottom from the point of view of educating future owners.

In practice we tend to see mongrels and moggies for vaccinations, random injuries such as cut pads, fight wounds, pulled muscles, road accidents and sickness brought on by raiding the bin or eating too many mice. We see pedigrees for all these things, too, but the vast majority of the time we see them for reasons of their breed and their breed alone. This has got to stop. I wanted to be a vet my whole life, but it is pedigree health issues that drove me out of practice. I spent all my time fixing man-made problems. I became sick and tired of being able to look at my day list and know what 90% of the animals would be coming in for just by what breed they were. The depressing reality didn't take long to sink in and now I'm writing this book again because things are getting worse, not better. I hope with all my heart that changes.

I will try to give you an insight into some of these diseases and the worst examples. I think the thing that upsets me most about inherited disease is that it has come about as a direct result of breeding for looks alone. By selecting for certain attributes that are visible on the exterior of the animal we have condensed the gene pool and ended up selecting for disease and weakness, too.

Although there are now many health schemes in place to eradicate these, as I said, they do not go far enough as yet and fundamentally, as we will discuss later, they are not mandatory. We should no longer see 'normal for breed' as an acceptable phrase. Unless it's normal for the majority of the healthy species it should simply not be tolerated and should be leapt on by the breed clubs and dealt with, no matter what the consequence for the look of the breed.

We have created a number of breeds that are simply non-viable. This may sound dramatic, but in many cases it's true. Without veterinary intervention some pedigree dogs and cats would not survive. We'll look at some of the body systems affected by inherited disease and the breeds worst affected, but this is not by any means going to be comprehensive. There is a fantastic book by Gough, Thomas and O'Neill (G, T and O) called *Breed Predispositions to Disease in Dogs and Cats*. It was completely updated in 2017 and if you have an interest in the extent of disease in our pedigrees then I strongly recommend it.

Heart Disease

As we mentioned in the last chapter, heart disease is a common cause of death in giant breeds. DCM being the major disease. But there are many other heart diseases that can affect cats and dogs. According to G, T and O, boxers are predisposed to six different heart conditions, DCM included. In fact, more than 90% of DCM cases are seen in purebred dogs.

However, when it comes to heart disease the Cavalier King Charles Spaniel is probably the breed most well-known for it. These dogs have been so very badly let down by their breed clubs and the Kennel Club. I know this is a generalisation and I know there are some wonderful people out there trying to do the right things for the breed, but it seems they are very much in the minority at the moment.

I have to say that I think Cavaliers are some of the best-natured dogs you will ever come across. I have never in 25 years of university and practice come across a single nasty one. This is pretty rare because there are usually one or two specimens of every breed that can be anything from a bit grumbly to downright savage. In a way the diseases these dogs get are made even sadder by the fact they're such lovely, sweet dogs, much like the Frenchies and pugs so appallingly afflicted with breed-related disease.

Cavaliers suffer from a type of heart disease called mitral valve disease (MVD). The disease is progressive and the affected valve undergoes changes over the life of the dog and a murmur develops. Heart valves should form a strong, blood-tight seal so that when the heart pumps blood it is pushed in one direction only. When valves in these dogs get diseased the seal is poor and blood can regurgitate in the wrong direction during the forceful beat. It is the noise of this regurgitation that can be heard as a murmur. The leaky valve decreases the efficiency of the heart and increases the workload on it. As time goes by the extra load causes changes throughout the heart and can lead to heart failure and early death. Half of Cavaliers will have a murmur by the age of five to seven years and almost *100%* will have a murmur by the age of ten. The KC 2014 health survey showed that around 38% of Cavaliers died from heart disease. One group campaigning vigorously for reform is Cavaliers Are Special. Their study reviews suggest that given that over two thirds of six-year-old cavaliers could have the SM we mentioned earlier and there is ample evidence that half of Cavaliers will have MVD by five to six years of age, it is likely that by seven years old more than half of them could have *both* conditions.

We are fortunate to live in a time in which we have excellent drugs to help with most conditions. Most drugs available for heart disease do not reverse or cure the condition, but they do prolong life and alleviate the symptoms. These drugs can make a big difference in some cases but the fact that medicine and surgery has come such a long way should not make it acceptable to continue breeding dogs with this level of disease. Just because we *can* fix something doesn't mean we should tolerate it as normal.

You can imagine my dismay when, as has often happened, I examine a six-year-old dog and say to the owner, 'Were you aware that she has a heart murmur?' and the owner says, 'Oh, yes, my last five of these died of heart failure. It is a problem, isn't it?' For goodness sake! This is another prime example of an abnormality being considered normal and acceptable. I'm constantly shocked by people repeatedly buying a breed when all their previous ones have been ill or died early!

The reason people don't stop buying them is that they are lovely dogs and many people have an affinity for a certain breed, and because we *know* Cavaliers die of heart disease and it's viewed as normal.

We'll talk more about health testing in the coming chapters, but suffice to say that while, in the UK, the life expectancy of these dogs has gone down in recent years, in Denmark, where they have introduced mandatory heart testing and protocols, they have seen a whopping 71% reduction in the risk of MVD.

And what about our lovely cats? While DCM is practically unheard of in cats, sadly, they do not escape heart disease. Cats tend to get something called hypertrophic cardiomyopathy, or HCM. Where the dogs get floppy, thin ventricle walls the cats go in the other direction. The walls of the heart become incredibly thickened and stiff and the volume of blood the ventricles can hold is vastly reduced. The end result is much the same – heart failure and death. It is seen most commonly in British shorthairs, Maine coons, Norwegian forest cats, Persians, ragdolls and the sphynx. The prevalence in the latter two is around 20%.

For all the breeders over the years that I've directly or indirectly come across there is one that stands out for me for all the right reasons. I had a lovely client who was a British shorthair breeder. She contacted the surgery one day and she was totally beside herself after finding one of her young stud cats dead in his enclosure; he had died of heart disease. This breeder immediately stopped breeding until she could afford to get every single breeding cat scanned. She also contacted every person that had ever had a kitten related to any of her affected cats. This should absolutely be the norm for anyone breeding animals, but sadly, in my experience, it is far from the case.

Skin Disease

We mentioned this in the skin chapter, but I want to put a little reminder here, too. Besides the conformation-related skin problems such as folds, atopic or allergic skin disease is definitely much more common in certain breeds than others. As we said, it usually starts at a young age and can mean a lifetime of misery for dogs and owners alike.

Westies are popular little dogs with very large personalities. In the 12 years before I left practice I saw very few Westies that did not have skin disease. I'm sure you'll remember the frighteningly graphic term 'armadillo Westies'. Some of the worst cases I've seen really have looked like this with thickened, black, wrinkled skin from years of chronic trauma. Some of the other breeds commonly affected are Labradors, golden retrievers, Dalmatians, Newfoundlands, German shepherd dogs, setters, some terriers, boxers and bulldogs.

Kidney and Bladder Problems

Many breeds of dogs and cats are prone to bladder crystals and stones. There are lots of different types of stones and they come about for different and complex reasons. Probably the most well-known case is the Dalmatian. Dalmatians have a metabolic defect that means they can't metabolise proteins in a normal way. Because of this they can have high levels of uric acid in their urine and this can lead to urate stone production. Bladder stones are a nuisance at best, but can, if they cause blockage and renal failure, be fatal. Other breeds prone to urates are bulldogs and Yorkies on the dog side and Bengals, Birmans, ragdolls, ocicats, Siamese, the sphynx and Egyptian maus on the cat side.

Some people have crossed Dalmatians with pointers and then bred them back to Dalmatians again. After a few generations you can't tell the difference in looks between a pure Dalmatian and one that had the pointer genes introduced. However, the back-crossed dogs have much lower levels of uric acid problems. It seems like a no-brainer to me!

Another inherited defect leading to stones and crystals called cystine is commonly seen in English bulldogs, Staffordshire bull terriers, Newfoundlands, mastiffs and dachshunds. Virtually all cases are seen in entire male dogs and in some cases neutering can help prevent the stones from recurring. My main job for the last several years has been as an advisor on medical nutrition. I spend a lot of time talking about the medical and dietary management of these stones. Sadly it is not uncommon to recommend neutering (most cases we get are bulldogs) and to get the reply from the vet that they have already discussed this and the owner has refused because they want to breed from the bulldog in question. It's also not unheard of at that point to find out that the dog is already on a different medical diet for its allergic skin disease!

A very difficult crystal and stone type to deal with is called calcium oxalate. Unlike some other types of bladder stones, this type can't be dissolved with medical or dietary management. Calcium oxalate stones can form with very few signs and also have a tendency to form inside the kidneys as well, which is even more of an issue when it comes to the outlook for these cases. Small breeds of dog such as terriers, miniature schnauzers, Lhasa apso and shih-tzus are most commonly reported, but there are also many breeds of pedigree cat as well, including Persians, Siamese, British and exotic shorthairs, Devon rex, Burmese and Scottish fold cats.

Sometimes calcium oxalate issues come hand in hand with renal disease and the poor old Persian suffers in this respect, too. Polycystic kidney disease (PKD) is a common inherited disorder in cats and can lead to death at a very young age. As it sounds, the kidneys have cysts that develop inside them and the normal, working tissue of the kidneys is gradually destroyed. Kidney cells, like brain cells, are never replaced and once the organs fail death is inevitable. Some breeds related to Persians have the same gene mutation. Other breeds most commonly affected are British and exotic shorthairs and the Himalayans.

There is no cure. Luckily nowadays we have medication and prescription diets that can help support the kidneys when they start to fail, but the bottom line is that this disease is a killer and all we can do with medicine is alleviate the symptoms and reduce the suffering. So, how much of a problem is it? You will probably be surprised to hear that the number of cats affected is around 40% across the world within the breeds affected. The gene that causes it is dominant, which means that even if only one parent has the gene, the chances are that half the litter will not only inherit the gene, but *will* have the disease. You can see how such a condition can become so prevalent so quickly.

For some time now there has been a scheme in place to try to screen for the condition. This consists of ultrasound scanning after ten months of age to look for the cysts, but there is also now a widely available genetic test that is very accurate for this type of PKD.

This is fantastic news because it means that breeders can make sure they don't breed from any affected cats. This is a sure-fire way to eradicate a disease where the inheritance is so fully understood. When I wrote my first book on pedigree health in 2007 the Governing Council of the Cat Fancy (GCCF), which is the cat equivalent of the Kennel Club, had a policy only to encourage breeders to do health tests. However, I'm *very* pleased to say that since 2016 it now makes it mandatory for Persian cats on the breeding register to be screened clear of PKD. What a huge step in the right direction.

A while ago a colleague of mine was talking to a Persian breeder about the disease and she was obviously concerned. He mentioned to her that screening was available and she was very keen to get it started and have her breeding cats scanned. However, once she realised the fact that she could potentially lose 50% of her available breeders she changed her mind and decided not to have the test done. This is not an uncommon scenario, no matter what the incidence of disease. Too often the look of the animal and its chance to do well at shows, and thus command good rates as a stud or for offspring, overrides the health of the animal. I've seen it many times and I believe it is wrong. By making health tests mandatory the governing bodies can set an example and lead the way for health and welfare. I hope they continue to do more.

That said, these disease rates do raise the valid question of even further reducing the gene pool by excluding affected cats from breeding and that is a real concern where things such as Persians and PKD are concerned. In order to get rid of the disease you have to exclude almost half the cats and may well end up with other disease problems because of even narrower breeding. I don't know what the answer is, but it seems to me that if a particular breed has such a level of potentially fatal, inherited disease we should consider whether to continue the breed at all.

A sensible step is out-crossing, as we said some people have done with the uric acid problem in Dalmatians. Many breeders are horrified at the idea of it. Outbreeding or outcrossing is as it sounds – the opposite of inbreeding. In effect it would mean letting another breed be introduced to a number of matings to try to dilute the genetic material of the breed and reduce the frequency of inherited disease. Breeders do not like the idea because it is seen as 'soiling' the purity of their blood lines. However, we are at a point where it may end up being the only option because the pool is fast turning into stagnant sludge and some fresh, running water is desperately needed.

As well as the cats, there are also some dog breeds with a higher than normal incidence of kidney disease. Boxers, Dobermanns, Cavaliers, cockers, English bull terriers and the Dogue de Bordeaux are all prone to kidney disease and sometimes an early death because of it.

Joint Disease and Skeletal Problems

As we have mentioned already in various places, there are many skeletal issues that are rife in some breeds. Some of this is due to their body shape, such as the bow-legged dogs and short-legged breeds including the dachshund and the dreadful Munchkin cat, but in others there are less easily explained diseases. The classic ones are hip dysplasia, elbow dysplasia and OCD. In many breeds such as the Labrador and German shepherd there is now a huge variation between working and show lines.

In 2017, just before the final of Crufts, there was a display given by the police dog handling team. It was brilliant as always. The difference in appearance and mobility between the police working dogs and the show shepherds was absolutely staggering; they had rumps high like racehorses and wild canids as opposed to the sloping disfigurement of the modern-day show shepherd. In Labradors as well it seems now that the chunky, squat show lines are almost unrecognisable as the same breed from their leggy, athletic working peers.

The fact is that working dogs have to be fit for purpose, they have a job to do so dogs with joint disease do not tend to get bred from. Buying from a working line may help avoid issues, but make sure you still ask about the tests that have hopefully been done. Also remember that working dogs need a huge commitment in time and energy to keep them stimulated.

Another breed that has had part of its skeleton drastically altered is the English bull terrier (see Figures 10.1 and 10.2). Many of you will know that this breed is famous for its 'Roman' nose. The breed standard says that viewed from the front the head and skull should be '… egg-shaped and completely filled, its surface free

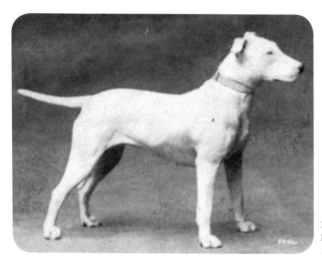

Figure 10.1: Bull terriers didn't have egg-shaped heads in the 1900s … (Photo: public domain)

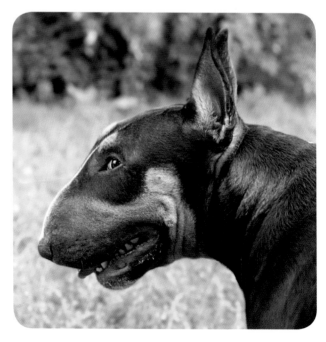

Figure 10.2: … unlike today. (Photo: Adobe Stock)

from hollows or indentations.' It goes on to say, 'Profile curves gently downwards from top of skull to tip of nose that should be black and bent downwards at the tip.'

This conformation is wildly different from a natural canid and, as so often happens, has a knock-on effect to other structures. The curving face with a downwards-pointing nose has changed the angles of the jaw bones and this means that the large canine teeth often do not erupt in the right position on the bottom jaw. They don't find the gap between the upper teeth where they should sit and instead end up inside the upper teeth, from where they will eventually eternally impinge on the hard palate. The selection for this skull shape is the cause of the majority of malocclusions (dental mismatches) in bull terriers.

Affected dogs will either have to have specialist dental procedures as the teeth erupt to reposition them or, if left too late, suffer the painful lesions you can see in Figures 10.3 to 10.5, and have the canine teeth extracted at a later date. Of course, the breed, like so many others, never used to look like this and has been markedly changed in the last few decades (see again Figures 10.1 and 10.2).

With skeletal issues we also have a tendency to actually select *for* abnormalities in certain breeds. Two such cases that come straight to mind are Rhodesian ridgebacks and Manx cats.

Manx cats are well known for their lack of tail. Some vary and have stubby, short tails, but many have no tail at all. Cats use their tails for balance and communication,

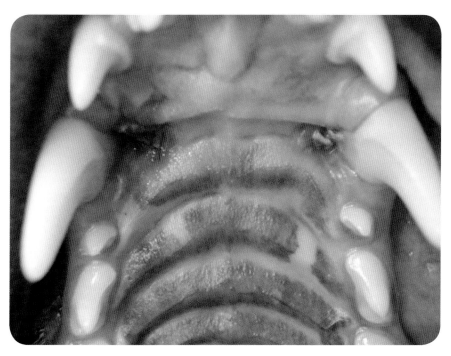

Figure 10.3: Painful holes in the hard palate from the lower canine teeth. (Photo: Jens Ruhnau)

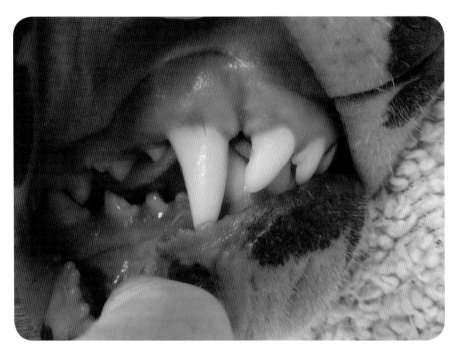

Figure 10.4: The bottom canines disappear inside the mouth because the jaw angle is wrong. (Photo: Jens Ruhnau)

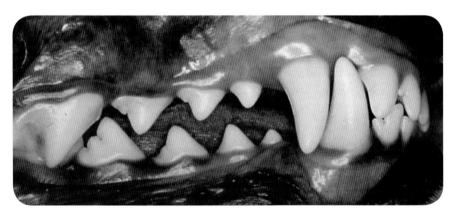

Figure 10.5: A normal mouth. (Photo: Dr Fraser Hale)

and it is totally unethical to breed cats without tails, but the lack of tail is not the biggest ethical problem with the continued, deliberate breeding of Manx cats. The defect that causes the short or absent tail is a spinal defect that causes varying degrees of spina bifida. It's a dominant inheritance, which means many kittens fail to develop and simply die in the womb. Those surviving will have varying degrees of spinal problems, from an odd gait through to faecal and urinary incontinence to arthritis and paralysis.

Apart from the issues that not having a tail has for the cats' movement and communication, I hope you will agree that effectively breeding *for* spina bifida can never be viewed as morally or ethically acceptable.

As for ridgebacks, the ridge is not as benign as it might seem. Ostensibly it is a ridge of hair that grows in the wrong direction down the spine of the dogs, giving them the characteristic ridge. In fact, the breed standard not only calls for a ridge, but very specifically defines it as follows;

A distinctive feature is the ridge on the back formed by hair growing in opposite direction to the remainder of coat. Ridge clearly defined, tapering and symmetrical, starting immediately behind shoulders and continuing to haunch, and containing two identical crowns only, opposite each other, lower edges of crowns not extending further down ridge than one third of its length.

So no mistaking the need for the presence of the ridge then!

In days gone by, and sometimes still in some countries, the puppies born without ridges were culled at birth. After *Pedigree Dogs Exposed* came out rules were passed in the UK that make it illegal to cull any animals for cosmetic reasons, but it does still go on elsewhere.

The genes that cause the ridge are also associated with something called a dermoid sinus. Dermoid sinuses are narrow, hollow tubes that lead from the skin to varying depths of the tissues underneath. This can lead to deep infections, but some sinuses actually go as deep as the spinal cord itself and can cause serious spinal infections, permanent problems and even death. The gene for the ridge is dominant so ridgeless dogs tend not to have sinus problems while puppies with two copies of the gene will be most at risk. One Swedish study showed that around 8–10% of ridged dogs are affected. Some sinuses can be removed surgically, but it is still commonplace for puppies born with sinuses to be culled.

In stark contrast to the breed standard, the Universities Federation for Animal Welfare (UFAW) website, another great resource for pedigree health information, has this to say;

This condition could possibly be eliminated by only breeding from ridge-less individuals. (At present, the breed standards, which are based on appearance not welfare considerations, specify that there should be a ridge). It is currently not known if the ridge-less population provides a large enough genetic pool for this to be carried out safely, within the breed, without narrowing the gene pool and exacerbating other genetically influenced conditions. It may therefore be necessary to outcross with other breeds in order to tackle this problem.

Quite clearly the continued breeding of ridged dogs is selecting for a developmental abnormality with potentially life-threatening consequences.

Intestinal Problems

As we mentioned in the giants chapter, some of the larger breeds are prone to GDVs, but there are many other intestinal problems for which some breeds definitely have a predisposition.

We see an increasing number of dogs these days with inflammatory bowel disease. Sometimes a cause is found, but many times we are left just trying supportive and dietary management. German shepherds, Rottweilers, Weimeraners, Yorkies and Border collies are among the most commonly reported breeds. Inflammatory bowel disease can lead to protein loss, and my sister's own beautiful Rottie cross, Ronnie, died at a young age because of intractable disease.

German shepherds also account for around 60% of cases of EPI; this stands for exocrine pancreatic insufficiency and it basically means they do not digest their food properly. They often appear thin despite eating ravenously and have fatty, greasy faeces. They can be very satisfying cases because usually a very good quality diet and supplements of pancreatic enzymes soon have many of them looking amazingly well.

Staying with the pancreas, we also now see increasing numbers of dogs with pancreatitis. This is a very serious inflammation of the pancreas and it can be fatal in severe cases. In dogs it is usually triggered by fatty foods, but some animals are much more sensitive than others. Cocker spaniels, miniature schnauzers and some terriers are the most commonly affected. This is very relevant in my line of work because some medical diets have high fat levels for other reasons and these diets can be very dangerous in certain breeds. Please don't buy medical or prescription diets online without speaking to your vet first!

The List Goes On ...

This is a tiny scratch on the surface of inherited disease. Suffice to say, you must do research! With more than 700 diseases recognised in pedigree dogs and cats there are certainly no guarantees. Some diseases are very rare, while others are rife in some breeds. Some may cause huge welfare issues, while others may be of passing academic interest only. For more information read Gough, Thomas and O'Neill, the UFAW website is excellent and also look at dogbreedhealth.com, which is also very comprehensive and being updated all the time.

As I've said many times, people rarely ask vets for advice before they buy. A depressing study recently found that people spend more time picking shoes than a dog! And we wonder why so many people are stunned when they end up with a diseased impulse buy. Don't be one of those people. PLEASE!

I think we'll finish this chapter with a reminder of part of that quote from UFAW,

'… the breed standards, which are *based on appearance not welfare* …'

Chapter 11

Designer Dogs, Moggies, Mutts and Mongrels

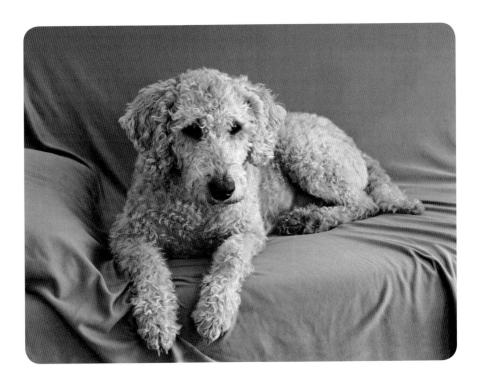

O NE OF MY MOST MEMORABLE CONSULTATIONS FROM ALL MY TIME IN practice was a first vaccination for a puppy. The practice I was working in split the time needed for these sessions between a vet and a nurse. I was seeing another client while Janet, the nurse, did her part of the puppy consultation in the room next door, covering preventative medicine such as worming and flea treatments, insurance, diet and so on before I arrived for the health exam and actual vaccination.

As I was writing up my previous notes she appeared in the doorway with a wry smile on her face. I said, 'What is it?' in a suspicious tone, not sure what to expect, fully knowing that she knew my views on pedigree health issues. She smiled, raised her eyebrows and said, 'Oh nothing. I'll just wait for you to come in.'

I scrutinised my screen to see what breed the puppy was to see if I could guess what was about to confront me and saw it just described on the computer as a cross-breed. I entered the room and saw the little black bundle on the consulting room table. On talking to the owner she told me in grave tones that she'd had a purebred boxer previously and it had had the most awful skin problems throughout its life. After such a horrible experience she had heard that cross-breeds were supposed to be healthier, so had decided to do the right thing and get a cross-breed. She had decided to get a basset hound crossed with a Shar-Pei!

If you cast your mind back to the previous chapters, I'm sure you'll realise that if you specifically set out to pick a cross between two breeds practically guaranteed to have skin disease you couldn't do better than this combination! To be fair the puppy was much less wrinkly than a Shar-Pei and had a more proportioned body and legs than a basset, so maybe she got lucky. In the end I moved practice before I got to find out.

The point is that, of course, there are, if you like, 50 shades of cross-breeds these days. When I was younger we phoned the RSPCA, got a list of unwanted dogs and ended up with a six-month-old mongrel called Penny. I was 11 and she was my faithful and healthy companion for 16 years. Back then there tended to be pedigrees and what we called Heinz 57s. I used this term recently and was shocked that the person to whom I was talking had not heard it. It means the dogs that are true mixes, the ones that you look at and you have no idea what on earth they are made up of. They are beautiful, individual, unique and generally robust animals.

So we know what pedigrees are, but it seems easy these days to get confused about what else is out there, especially with the fairly recent advent of the designer cross-breeds.

Mongrels, Mutts, Moggies and Doggies

As we said all the way back at the beginning, the word pedigree conjures up images of grandeur and noble ancestry. Conversely, for some reason, mongrels are some-times seen in exactly the opposite way. I have long pondered this and the reason. What is it that drives us to want a certain breed of dog or cat? Almost certainly their physical characteristics that we find attractive, or that suit our lifestyle, or that we want to parade in front of our friends, but there is also this myth that you know what you're getting.

In the KC meeting I mentioned before about the police German shepherds I was told, unforgettably once again, that the priorities for breeders, in this order, were 1) looks, 2) temperament and 3) health. Again, I was lost for words. I thought to

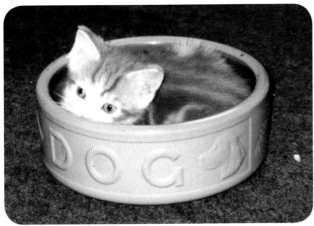

Figures 11.1, 11.2, 11.3, 11.4: Some of the beautiful moggies and mutts that have graced our lives.

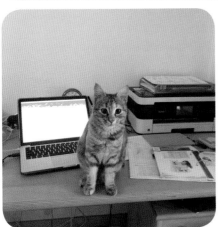

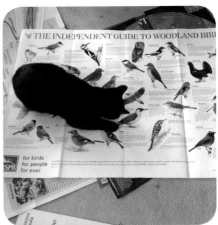

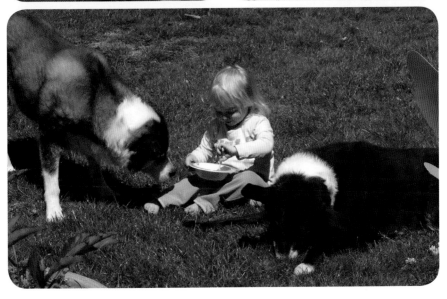

myself I must be mistaken. Surely he didn't mean in *that* order so I asked specifically if that's what he meant. Yes.

I said I found it shocking that anyone would openly say that they cared more about looks than health, to which he replied, 'Well, we don't want a load of dogs going round biting everyone.' People whose arguments don't hold up often try misdirection to deflect people from their failed attempts to defend a position. Of course, temperament is important, as important for a family pet as health, but looks should never be placed above these.

So, people feel that if they pick a pedigree they will be able to predict its temperament and behaviour. Of course, this is true to a degree because we have selected dogs for certain characteristics, but there are two things I find difficult with this. Firstly, it's a dangerous assumption to make and secondly, why does it imply that a mongrel would have a worse temperament than a pedigree?

Let's look at the first point – the danger of the assumption. If you speak to any vets that have been in practice for any length of time they will have all been attacked at some point by a surprising patient. Most vets will have certain breeds of which they are wary. For me, I was most suspicious of Jack Russells and other terriers, Border collies, German shepherds and mastiffs. I'm not being 'breedist', it's just that these were the breeds that were most likely to try to bite me. It was my own personal experience. *But*, I have also been viciously attacked by Labradors and retrievers, to name but a few. The danger was that it was more unexpected because they are breeds that many people view as sweet, family dogs.

No one should ever assume that any dog is 100% safe or otherwise; it will depend on a million things. The danger comes when people assume, as many do, that, for example, all Labradors make perfect family pets and you can let your kids do anything you like to them. You can't. Animals need space and respect and the number of videos that circulate on social media showing children hugging, gripping, pulling, riding and crawling on dogs sends fear through every vet and behaviour specialist because they are accidents waiting to happen.

When people tell me they want a French bulldog or a Cavalier because their temperament is so good it breaks my heart. The majority of dogs on the planet could have a lovely temperament, that's why we like them! We just need to pick the right puppies and kittens and give them the best start in life. The temperament of some dogs is hugely affected by chronic pain and disease, so surely by choosing less diseased specimens we will already be improving our chances of having a happy, well-natured pet? If we properly outlawed puppy farms at home and abroad we could ensure better socialised and habituated animals.

In practice I never felt fearful of a mongrel the way I did about certain other breeds, which comes to my second point. Why do we assume that mongrels will be somehow unpredictable or inferior to a pedigree equivalent? It's backwards and it's a psychological mismatch that we need to address. It feels almost racist, another facet of human nature that I can't abide. As I said, temperament depends on a multitude of factors and I'll give you some pointers for that in a later chapter. For now, try to wipe assumptions about temperament, good and bad, from your mind.

So maybe mongrels are seen as the peasantry to the nobility of the pedigrees, but actually the way we need to start to view true mongrels and moggies (the cat equivalent) is as champions of random chance and hybrid vigour.

Hybrid vigour, according to the *Oxford Living Dictionary*, is, 'The tendency of a cross-bred individual to show qualities superior to those of both parents.' What a great definition for something nature does unwittingly. It's described as the opposite of inbreeding depression where offspring of related parents are less fit because of accumulation of recessive genes. Mongrels and moggies are, quite clearly, the way forward!

I've long pondered why moggies are so much more popular than mongrels. I think it's partly because cats have always been the same. The vast majority of people just want a cat; they don't make a distinction in their head. They might prefer a certain colour or a certain hair length, but the animal inside is just a cat. I truly wish we could go back to seeing dogs the same way. I used the word doggie in the title of this section. It makes me cringe when used in the normal way when people speak to toddlers as if they're idiots and point out the nice 'doggie', but I think we should reclaim the word. The dog equivalent of a healthy, robust moggie; the doggie! I think it could really take off.

There's another major difference between doggies and moggies, certainly, in the Western world, and that is availability. For decades we have tackled the problem of stray animals by neutering all and sundry. This is hugely important for the welfare of the wider population of animals that never find a home, but it has had a big impact on the number of true mongrels you can find. Semi-feral cats remain an issue so the supply of hybrid, healthy moggies is still pretty unaffected.

I am a huge fan of adoption. Dogs in adoption centres are often seen as damaged individuals, but many of them are there for reasons of circumstance such as divorce, death and financial issues. For me these centres are brilliant sources of beautiful mongrels, but increasingly they are filling up with pedigree outcasts and rejects; dogs taken on because of a fashionable whim only for the owners to realise the devastating health issues. Adoption organisations are also now having to cope with the tide of puppies being illegally imported from Europe to meet the huge demand for pedigree dogs in the UK and beyond, something that hopefully the law will soon start to tackle. Our obsession with breeds of dog is having a serious knock-on effect. If we started outcrossing and breeding for true health, not looks, we'd have a very different population of animals.

Back in 2008 I did some work in South Africa with the fantastic organisation International Fund for Animal Welfare (IFAW). We visited the townships around Cape Town and Johannesburg to help raise awareness and try to encourage vets to volunteer there. The trip was pretty harrowing with humans and animals alike living in extreme poverty, the like of which most of us can't begin to imagine. The dogs we treated there were malnourished and riddled with parasites, but they were strong, inherently healthy individuals (see Figures 11.5–11.8). They

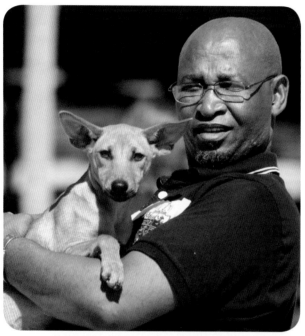

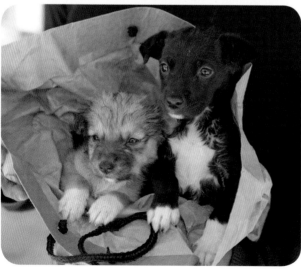

Figures 11.5, 11.6, 11.7, 11.8: Unique, robust and beautiful mongrels from my trip with IFAW. (Photo: IFAW)

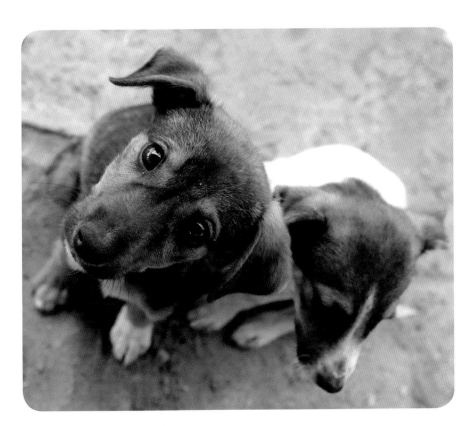

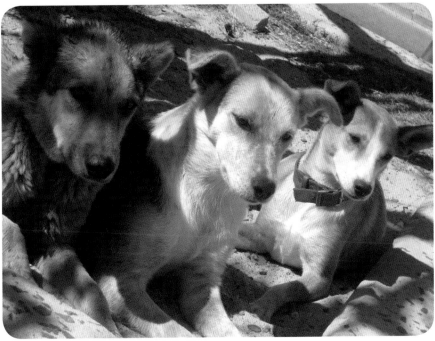

have to be to survive. They were medium-sized, short-haired, dog-shaped dogs. They were products of random breeding and survival of the fittest. Put one of our extremes or inbreds there? No chance.

My husband is a wind fanatic and we've spent a lot of time in a wild and beautiful part of Spain called Tarifa. I absolutely love going there. When we go for sundowners, it's absolute chaos! There are children and dogs everywhere, all running free. It's what many of us would consider totally irresponsible, but because of the culture the dogs are amazingly well socialised, they are free from leads that often cause frustration and aggression and they are habituated to kids from the word go. And virtually all of them are mongrels. We occasionally see holidaymakers there with precious pedigrees on a lead, desperate to play but never allowed, but on the whole the local dogs are a collection of robust mongrels, all individual and wonderfully varied in appearance.

It's a big social question how we would go about even considering returning to out-crossed, healthier dogs, but it's something we need to tackle now, not in another ten years' time.

Designer Cross-breeds

What a fly in the ointment these have been. Sadly, as pedigree health has deteriorated, just as my basset–Shar-Pei owner thought, people have ended up being tempted into buying animals called cross-breeds that are very little to do with true mongrels or hybrid vigour.

In genetic terms, designer cross-breeds are called F1 crosses. They are the first cross of two distinct parent types. The absolute classic is the Labradoodle. These crosses between, as you can guess, Labradors and poodles became extremely popular in the late 1980s and are still highly regarded. Breeders often say they are hypoallergenic, so people who suffer allergies to dogs can have them. This is not true; some may be better for some people, but no animals are hypoallergenic. As we said before, allergies are not usually to fur on animals, but to dander or skin fragments. Animals that shed less fur may be preferable for some people, but the cross is no guarantee of zero allergic reaction.

The Labradoodle epitomises the problem with designer cross-breeds and the poor messaging it sends out. You take two breeds with significant health concerns, you mix them together and your result will be a total lottery. In practice I have seen labradoodles that have won the genetic lottery and avoided the joint disease of the Labrador and the skin disease of the poodles, but equally my husband and I have seen the puppies that have inherited the whole shebang, one of which was euthanased at six months of age due to terrible health.

Cockapoos, cavapoos, puggles and numerous other F1 crosses are springing up now, the major disadvantage being that the parent gene pools are already so small there remains a high chance that the puppies will not be healthier than the parents. Hybrid vigour certainly won't be guaranteed by crossing two diseased individuals.

In fact, Wally Conron, the Australian breeder credited with 'inventing' the Labradoodle, has since said he regrets having done it. The craze for designer crosses since the Labradoodle has led to more health problems, unscrupulous breeders and abandoned animals, rather than generally improved health. If you're looking for a cross-breed, get a mutt, mongrel, moggie or doggie. Paying a grand or two for a designer cross when you could adopt a true mix is absolute madness.

One final word on designer crosses; the F1 cross that would sum up my thoughts on these would have to be a bulldog crossed with a shih-tzu. I'm sure you can work out what it would be called!

So now you are armed with the facts about the unhealthy among us it's time to look at how you can go about choosing a healthy and *happy* puppy or kitten. Dogs and cats are pretty different in some ways and you're probably choosing one or the other, so to save you finding the relevant bits we'll split them into two. Dogs, then cats. There's some things that apply to both, but don't worry, I'll repeat word-for-word what's necessary so you don't need to read both chapters to get all the information you need.

Chapter 12

How to Choose a Healthy Puppy

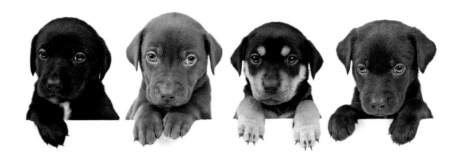

A s with everything in life, there are no guarantees. There will be those of you out there who have had a cross-breed with poor health and, of course, there are plenty of pedigree animals that breeze through life with no issues at all. Equally, with the other tips in this chapter they are generalisations; pointers to try and make sure that you avoid the most common pitfalls when it comes to picking a puppy. No one step will guarantee a healthy dog, but if you follow all the steps you've got a much higher chance of having a healthy, well-adjusted pet.

Before we get started, first and foremost, I'd like you to consider adoption. Whether you decide to go for a pedigree or not please remember that there are thousands of animals in adoption centres that need homes; they are not all tainted goods. Even if you think you're sure you know what you want why not just go and have a look? You've got nothing to lose and possibly everything to gain. The good organisations do excellent behavioural assessments and they can also help you match dogs to your lifestyle and family circumstances. You never know, you might just fall in love. There's no obligation and you can always walk away. It's also wise to consider an older animal from an adoption centre; puppies can be a huge pain in the bum! By taking on an older animal you can avoid the chewing, house-training and the unruly adolescent years. You'll also be making the life of an older animal vastly better.

Some lovely people in the village we used to live in went to the local adoption centre convinced of what sort of dog they wanted and came back with the exact opposite because they were simply destined for each other. If you're desperate for a pedigree then think about breed-specific adoption, there are plenty of those, too. All I ask is that before you ring someone for the instant gratification puppy online you spend a few hours one afternoon wandering along the aisles of your local adoption centre. Do it for me and if you find something you love let me know on Twitter or Facebook. I'd love to hear about it and, of course, see some photos.

Before you get a Puppy or Dog

So now let's get down to business and the first thing we need to tackle is YOU! One of the biggest causes of abandonment of animals, dogs especially, is owners making the wrong choices. This can be because of breed ill health and unexpected costs, so hopefully I've armed you with the facts in the previous chapters to avoid the worst of those. We'll be looking more clearly at that soon as well. Besides ill health, though, many owners pick animals based on a whim or a fashion. A film called *Sled Dogs* came out years ago, and *Game of Thrones* has recently caused another surge in impulse buying of huskies. Huskies have had running *drilled* into their DNA. Unless you are a high-performance athlete with no job you are unlikely to have the time and energy to truly meet the needs of a husky. St Bernards became hugely popular after the film *Beethoven* and I shudder to think what the fallout from the poorly conceived film *Patrick: Pug... Actually* will be! A glamorous celebrity is photographed with a minuscule Chihuahua in a handbag and the process continues.

Different breeds of dog can be *so* different in their characteristics that they are almost like different species. You need to understand the needs of the dog you are taking on and be *totally honest* with yourself about your situation. This sounds like a blatant plug, and it is, but please consider my *Pet Detective* series to help your research. They are aimed at children, but are great for adults, too. With chapters on each of the five welfare needs and the wild ancestors/relatives to help understand how the animals like to live, they are a useful tool for knowing if any dog is suitable for you. There is also a virtual month for your children or you to complete to give you a taster of what being a dog owner is all about.

The Five Welfare Needs

I mentioned the five welfare needs there and I hope that you are all familiar with them, but surveys every year suggest that many pet owners are still in the dark about these terms. The welfare needs form the basis of the Animal Welfare Act 2006 in England and Wales, the Scottish Animal Health and Welfare Act 2006 and also the Northern Ireland Welfare of Animals Act 2011. The needs are also a brilliant, simple way to approach the care of any animal in the world, captive or wild. By law, in the UK and in many other countries it is your duty of care to provide for these needs and if you don't you could be prosecuted. Even in places where it isn't the law I believe it is our moral duty to provide for our pets. I've always said that having a pet is a privilege, not a right. Just because you want one doesn't mean you should have one if you can't keep it happy and healthy. The health side of the needs are, in some ways, the easiest to get right. The happiness needs are much more difficult, but *so* important for both the mental wellbeing of your dog and the likelihood of it fitting into your blissful domestic situation!

We'll look at the needs here because it's a good way for you to start to think about your house, life and relationships and how your dog might fit in.

I'll give you a few basic pointers about the needs, but this book is more about picking your pet than looking after it once you've got it. Please listen to your veterinary team and ask them about other respected sources of post-purchase advice. The needs are all intertwined, of course, but I see the first three needs listed here as health and the last two as happiness:

1. **The need for a suitable diet and fresh water.** Dogs (apart from puppies up to weaning) don't need anything else to drink except water. Fresh water should be available all the time. Depriving animals, especially puppies, of water at night or various times to help with such things as toilet training is cruel and dangerous. Please get behavioural advice rather than risk dehydration.

    When it comes to food, there are about a million choices. Which you pick will be your choice and will likely be dictated by things including your finances and your sources of information, hopefully one of which will be your vet. In general the more expensive the food, the better quality and the more controlled/quality-checked it will be. 'Open formula' foods are cheaper and their ingredients may change from batch to batch; for the majority of animals this is fine. Fixed formula foods are more expensive and the ingredients are guaranteed to be the same from batch to batch unless there is an upgrade of some kind. Make sure whatever food you feed is complete and balanced.

    Dogs are omnivores like humans and evolved alongside us eating our scraps. They have been proven to have the genes necessary for digesting carbohydrates, some of which wolves do not have. Dogs are *not* wolves and can't be fed like them. The latest craze for grain-free foods for dogs is unnecessary. Grain intolerance in dogs is incredibly rare, just as it is in humans. Grains are a very important source of many types of beneficial fibre and vitamins.

Do not feed raw meats. It presents a significant public health risk, not just to your dog but to you, your family and the wider population of animals and humans. Home cook food if you want to, but don't feed raw.

Be aware that puppies need higher energy foods with certain ratios of phosphorous and calcium for healthy growth and joints. They also need specific fatty acids for optimal brain and eye development. I would urge you to feed your puppy a quality, complete puppy food recommended by your vet. If, as an adult, your dog is likely to weigh more than 25kg they need a large breed puppy food to reduce the risk of growth abnormalities.

Don't be shy about money. You need to work out how much your dog is likely to eat as an adult and decide if you can afford to feed him or her for hopefully 15 years or more.

Finally, ask your vet about body condition score, or BCS. This is how to assess if your puppy is the right weight. Obesity is a massive problem now, with many people perceiving fat animals as the right weight. Keep your puppy slim, get into good habits from the word go and they are more likely to stay slim for life, be healthier and live longer.

2.   **The need for a suitable environment.** For dogs this just means your home, but your home might not be suitable for any dog let alone the sort of dog you might think you want. Find out the energy and exercise needs of the breed or size of dog that you are thinking of getting. If you don't have a garden, think carefully about whether you can be bothered to go for walk six to ten times a day so your dog can have a wee and a poo. And that's on top of its actual exercise. You'll need to look at the cost of beds, toys, bowls, collars, leads and replacing them. You need to think about where your dog will go when it is muddy and wet from a walk. Will it be allowed in your bedroom at night? Will you let it on the furniture? Is your house like a show home and do you want it covered in hair, dribbled water, half-chewed things and mud? Because if your dog is to be happy your house will be covered in these things!

3.   **The need to be protected from pain, injury and disease.** Veterinary medicine has grown and developed at a similar rate to human medicine. We have the same drugs, surgical equipment, levels of sterility, surgical expertise and medical evaluation, and imaging equipment from a basic X-ray machine to a state-of-the-art MRI scanner. Vets are expensive; that is a fact of modern life. It's not because we are thieving money-grabbers, it's because this stuff costs a lot of money and to ensure the gold standard of care for your pet we have highly trained staff who deserve to be paid for their expertise. People in the

UK are used to what appears to be free healthcare for themselves, so we resent paying for care for our animals. As I said, having an animal is a privilege not a right. You need to very carefully consider how much your dog's veterinary care might cost from the most basic vaccination or consultation up to the costs of major surgery should it be needed.

The excellent charity the PDSA produces a yearly report into pet ownership in the UK called the PAW report. It makes for very interesting reading and is readily available online. Around three-quarters of owners underestimate the lifetime costs of owning a dog. The minimums, depending on the size of the dog according to the 2017 report are between £6,500 and £17,000. The report goes on to say that these are minimums and that for some dogs it could be as high as a whopping £33,000. None of these sums is insignificant, so think carefully about your finances before you take on a puppy.

As for preventing disease, vets recommend vaccination and effective parasite control because it helps keep your pets safe, alive and comfortable; it's not because we are villains! Please vaccinate your puppy and let it continue on into adulthood. The raging conspiracy theories about vaccination in the human and animal world are dangerous scaremongering and are leading to preventable deaths of animals, children and adults; it's like going back to the Dark Ages. Vaccines save lives. Fact. We all need to be concerned about over-vaccination, but good vets will split vaccines and only give the ones that are necessary. Vaccines are different for different diseases and produce varying lengths of immunity. Some of these need to be given yearly, some don't. Don't listen to the loons saying that animals don't need vaccines. Trust me, I have seen at first-hand dogs die of diseases such as parvovirus and leptospirosis and it is a horrific way to go. The World Small Animal Veterinary Association (WSAVA) has excellent information about vaccination and it's produced by the leading veterinary experts in the world. If you're concerned about vaccination have a read of the website.

Do not use homeopathic vaccines, or any homeopathic remedies for that matter. They are unscientific, unproven and ineffective.

4. **The need to be kept with or without other animals.** The first of our happiness needs and such an important one. Humans are social animals, even if we don't seem like it sometimes, and so are dogs. They don't have to live with dog company, they can make do with us too, but they don't like being left alone. Some will cope, some definitely won't, but even the ones that cope and seem 'fine' or 'happy' alone will be unhappy and possibly frustrated or frightened. If you are going to be out all day at work, or even nip home for lunch and to give your dog a pat on the head and whizz out for a pee, you should not get a

dog. It's not acceptable for a dog to be left alone for long periods of time. Be honest with yourself and do the right thing. Some pets can be happy on their own, so rethink your choices.

5. **The need to behave normally.** Here's an extract from my kids' book on dogs about what normal dogs do. Normal dogs 'Poo, wee, whine, bark, howl, sniff each other's bums, chase animals, play bow, steal food, vomit and then eat it again, watch another dog vomit and then eat it, chew everything, bite, scratch, dig up your garden, shed hair, slobber, eat messily, bury toys in your sofa cushions, roll in fox poo, jump in muddy streams, shake the mud from streams all over you and your car, jump up at strangers, bark at the postman, bark at the door, bark at men in helmets, bark at passing cars and, of course, bark at the moon!'

Dog behaviour is a minefield and we'll look a little bit at it later, but dogs, puppies in particular, can drive you mental and they are a huge commitment. Lots of dogs are very trainable and training your dog can be fun and stimulating for both of you and help you bond. Having a well-behaved dog transforms your life and means you'll be able to go to so many more places with your dog. However, this need isn't about training, it's about letting animals be animals. Dogs have an innate need to interact, play, run, sniff, explore, chase, herd and all manner of other things that evolution and domestication have drilled into them. It's not OK to deprive an animal of one of its needs because it is inconvenient to us. Exercise is massively important to dogs and it is one of the things we deprive them of most. Often they are too badly behaved to go off the lead and more often we are too lazy or busy to walk them. It's not acceptable. I would strongly suggest that if you think you want a dog you go for at least half an hour's walk at least twice a day, *every single day* for a month. Weather must make no difference, you have to go. It's a lot harder than you think and you need to do that every day for 15 years. Try it for me.

The PDSA PAW report in 2017 found that 13% of dogs (1.2 *million* dogs) have had no training at all, **93,000** dogs NEVER get walked and a third of dogs only get one walk a day. This is a travesty for animal welfare and I hope you won't be that sort of owner. Lack of exercise and stimulation are a major cause of obesity and frustration, and also contribute to dog bite injuries. Getting out with your dog is great for both of you, so do it!

Well, now we've dealt with you we need to start your puppy-picking process. Right from the start let's start to narrow your choices for the good of dog-kind and talk about the elephant in the room straight away; breed health.

Breed Health

I know this whole book so far has been about this, but we need to crystallise that information. Now I know this is going to get me a whole load of abuse from lovers of certain breeds, but I'm not writing this book for them, I'm writing it for people who have an open mind and care deeply about the health of their future beloved pet and want to make the right decision. The title of this book is *Picking a Pedigree?*, but actually I've been a bit sneaky because I don't want you to pick a pedigree! In general you are more likely to get a healthy animal if you pick a true hybrid cross-breed. At the moment, until we start breeding for health not looks, all pedigrees by the nature of inbreeding will be more likely to be ill than a mongrel.

What comes next is my personal opinion, but I hope I have backed it up with the information in the book. I'm going to list below the breeds that, at this time, I would strongly urge you *not* to buy, either because of extremes of conformation (body shape) or because of high levels of inherited disease. In these breeds, if you do decide to go ahead please find out about health testing and do *not* accept a puppy from a breeder that doesn't test and openly share the results. There are good breeders out there, just make sure you find one. If you ignore me on the extremes of body shape then good luck! Obviously, I hope that time will change these breeds into less extreme, healthier versions of themselves, so keep an eye out because in another 20 years this list might be very different. I hope it will be non-existent, but I've been hoping that for the last 20 years! I must for balance point out that there are, of course, many individuals of these breeds that have had no health issues at all. I'm steering you away from these breeds because I believe that they are the most affected on the whole, so if you avoid them you are already ahead of the game when it comes to your chances of a healthy companion. Also, bear in mind that different breeds have different diseases in various countries because of different gene pools, so check what's most relevant in your area of the world.

Breeds to avoid	Reason
American cocker spaniel	Extreme conformation and inherited disease
Basset bleu	Extreme conformation
Basset hound	Extreme conformation
Boston terrier	Extreme conformation and brachycephalic
Boxer	Brachycephalic and inherited disease
Bulldog	Extreme conformation, brachycephalic and inherited disease
Bull mastiff	Extreme conformation, brachycephalic and inherited disease
Bull terrier (English)	Extreme conformation

Cavalier KCS	Extreme conformation, brachycephalic and inherited disease
Chihuahua	Extreme conformation and inherited disease
Chinese Crested	Hairless
Chow chow	Extreme conformation and inherited disease
Clumber spaniel	Extreme conformation
Corgi (all types)	Extreme conformation
Dachshund (all types)	Extreme conformation
Dandie Dinmont	Extreme conformation
Dobermann	Inherited disease
Dogue de Bordeaux	Extreme conformation, brachycephalic and inherited disease
French bulldog	Extreme conformation and brachycephalic
German shepherd dog	Inherited disease
Great Dane	Inherited disease
Griffon Bruxellois	Extreme brachycephaly
Irish wolfhound	Inherited disease
Japanese chin	Extreme brachycephaly
King Charles spaniel	Extreme conformation, brachycephalic and inherited disease
Mastiff	Extreme conformation and inherited disease
Neapolitan mastiff	Extreme conformation and inherited disease
Newfoundland	Inherited disease
Pekingese	Extreme brachycephaly
Pomeranian	Extreme conformation
Pug	Extreme brachycephaly and conformation
Rottweiler	Inherited disease
Skye terrier	Extreme conformation
Shar-Pei	Extreme conformation and inherited disease
Shih-tzu	Brachycephaly
St Bernard	Inherited disease

The fact is that I've listed around 30 breeds here, which seems a lot, but I've still left you with more than 150 other breeds to choose from if you want a pedigree dog. Choose carefully, mind, because these are just the worst affected; the others can still have problems.

As I said, this list will evolve with time and different countries' animals have slightly different disease lists because their genetic pools are different; the extremes of conformation are not greatly affected by region. There are some breeders pushing for the return to previous versions of some of the extreme breeds. Genetic screening has made a big difference to the health of some breeds and there are lots of people working towards positive change. I've listed these breeds because humans have a tendency to like quirky-looking things, but by making dogs look quirky we have undoubtedly made them diseased and the future buyers are the key to reducing the demand for these animals. Please try not to be influenced by celebrities and their fashionable breeds or social media hype. The current global adulation for brachycephalics is mirrored with equally *negative* feelings from vets, nurses and welfare organisations. Listen to the professionals, not Instagram and the like!

Remember to look back at the beautiful wild canids and cross-breeds from round the world. Whatever dog you look at, be it in a book, online or at an adoption centre, try to pick a dog that is roughly dog-shaped, in proportion, wrinkle-free and with appendages that are not giant or tiny! Put your trust in Mother Nature and evolution, not the modern-day Frankensteins looking to create beings at their whim.

Breed Characteristics

As I've already mentioned, you can't judge all animals in a breed as identical when it comes to predicted temperament, which is why the ridiculous Dangerous Dogs Act is one of the biggest disasters of animal legislation ever. *But*, as I said in the section about you, there are certain differences in general that we have to consider when picking an animal. We've selected dogs for herding, guarding and hunting over many, many years and these instincts are deep in their DNA. This means that some breeds will have more of a tendency to certain behaviours than others. Many vets will have seen Border collies herding their families into the consulting room! This may not always be an issue, but you need to think carefully about your home situation, energy levels, social life and working life.

An animal's behaviour is influenced by its genes and its environment. In the case of dogs, that environment is largely early life experiences (what we call socialisation and habituation), which we'll be getting to shortly. Good socialisation, habituation and puppy training can help fill in some of the flaws in behaviour left by their genes, but not always. In the case of a dog's temperament, in particular, it is as if their genes acting as a 'ceiling' beyond which no amount of socialisation will make a real difference. It's not all in 'how you raise them'; their genes still have a lot to answer for!

There is an optimum time for socialisation to happen and that is from three weeks old until somewhere in the region of 12–18 weeks old, with breeds such as huskies and the herding breeds appearing to finish this period sooner rather than later. Dogs do not reach full social maturity until one to three years of age and during this time their genes, as well as their environment, continue to affect their temperament. A classic example of this is the Staffie that is beautifully socialised and habituated as a puppy, but by the time he is three years old has turned into the Staffie stereotype – great with people, but tricky with other dogs. It's really important to look at the history of any breed that you are considering.

A major cause of relinquishment is people choosing dogs that are really inappropriate for their situation. Vets often see these poor choices, such as elderly owners, or busy families, taking on very lively dogs, herding dogs, or dogs from a working background. Herding and/or working collies, Labradors, retrievers, pointers, spaniels and the like will have enormous physical exercise and mental stimulation needs, which need to be met *every day*. This may well not make them ideal family pets. Be aware also that retrieving breeds can have a higher than average tendency to guard possessions, despite their otherwise amiable nature.

On this note please, don't follow the mad craze recently of importing and 'rescuing' street dogs from places such as Romania. This may seem noble, but from a behaviour and temperament point of view is fraught with difficulty and the chances of you getting a dog that isn't fearful and aggressive and doesn't guard its resources fiercely after life on the streets is slim. Also, more importantly the money it costs you could do way more in the dog's original country if donated, and we have plenty of dogs here needing homes.

You also need to read breed descriptions carefully and recognise the 'estate agent'-style language. For example, many of the traditional guarding or fighting breeds are perhaps described as 'loyal', 'aloof' or 'discerning with people'. This actually translates into 'difficult to socialise and aggressive with strangers'. You may think you want a dog that dislikes strangers, but remember the dog will not discriminate between strangers you like or know and those that you don't!

There is a huge variety within each breed for genetic make-up, but these tendencies will be there to some degree. You can do lots with good habits, training and socialisation, but some of your future dog's personality will be fixed by its genes. Temperament is everything, so picking animals with parents that have great temperaments is absolutely essential. No one should be breeding *any* dogs that are fearful or aggressive.

Finding a Good Breeder for Any Dog, Not Just Pedigrees

Adopt, adopt, adopt, adopt, adopt. Just saying! But if you are going to pick a pedigree from a breeder there are things you *must* know. At the time of writing in the UK and abroad we have huge problems with puppy farms and imported puppies from other puppy farms. Breeding is almost entirely unregulated. You can have a puppy within a day if you want one and you can still buy puppies in shops, which really makes you wonder if we are a nation at the forefront of animal welfare or not. We live in an era in which people are used to having something the instant they decide they want it. As I said before, a recent study found that people spend more time picking shoes than a dog. This is madness. View getting an animal like getting married or having a tattoo done. You definitely shouldn't rush into any of them! If you're being pestered by your kids for a puppy, please buy them the *Pet Detective* book I mentioned and get them to do the work for you.

So what's the issue with puppy farms, here and abroad? Everything! Dogs are sentient beings, not machines for profit. Breeding adults have a right to a good life and having their needs met. Puppy farm dogs live in absolutely squalid conditions and are completely isolated. They have none of their most basic needs met, including adequate food and water. The puppies they produce have poor immunity, multiple health problems and are not socialised or habituated. We'll be talking more about socialisation later, but believe me; you don't want a puppy that has spent its most formative weeks in a cage on a puppy farm.

Puppies being imported illegally into the UK are a huge issue now. The breeders say they have passports, but a passport can't be issued until the animal has been vaccinated against rabies and they can't have a rabies vaccination until 12 weeks of age. This means if someone is advertising a puppy with a passport and it's under 12 weeks of age, either they are lying about its age, or its vaccination status, or both. Puppies can't travel abroad for another 21 days after being vaccinated either, which means any properly vaccinated puppy will be at least 15 weeks old before it gets to you. As you now know, this may well be past its critical socialisation period, and you will never have any idea of the dog's parents or where it was raised.

Puppy sales are for organised crime now on the same scale as drug dealing. There is a great deal of money to be made, so the dealers go to extraordinary lengths to appear legitimate. They even have mocked-up houses where they show the puppy with what is claimed to be the mother because of the success of campaigns such as Where's Mum?, which encourage people not to buy puppies without seeing the mother. This can make it very hard for people looking for a good breeder.

Puppy farms and dealers often have multiple breeds of dogs, so never pick a breeder advertising multiple breeds. Try and look for photos of the puppies with the mother in a home setting, not puppies sitting against a generic backdrop.

The RSPCA website is an excellent resource and has these tips for how to spot dodgy dealers' adverts online:

Read adverts carefully and look out for the telltale signs:

- Dealers may use the same contact number on more than one advert. Try Googling the number to see if it has been used on any other puppy adverts.
- Descriptions may have been copied and pasted to be used on more than one advert – try Googling the description and see if it has been used before, word-for-word.

- Words such as 'miniature' and 'teacup' can be a sign of dealers trying to capitalise on popular terms.
- Photos of the puppies may have been used on other adverts. Right-click on the photo, select 'search Google for image' and see if it has been used on other ads.
- If the advert says a puppy has been vaccinated – check how old he or she is. A puppy cannot be vaccinated before four–six weeks of age. So, if a person is advertising a three-week-old vaccinated puppy, they are lying.
- If the puppy is advertised as having a passport, it has most probably been imported.
- We have seen dealers claim they are Kennel Club registered to convey legitimacy, but be wary of this. Ask for original documents and check with the Kennel Club before buying a puppy.
- Promises of 'free insurance' and 'puppy packs' do not mean the advert is from a legitimate breeder.

One of the biggest reasons that puppy farms continue is the sympathy factor. I'm constantly amazed that some people will still arrange to meet someone in places such as motorway services to buy a puppy. Please never, ever get a puppy without seeing where it was raised. Puppies are adorable whatever state they're in, and even when people see an unhealthy looking puppy they feel sorry for it, so they buy it to 'save' it. Sadly, all this does is perpetuate the demand and the suffering of the animals being used to produce these puppies. *Do not* buy an unhealthy puppy because you feel sorry for it. Tell the breeder/dealer they should be ashamed of themselves, walk away and report the advert/mobile number to the RSPCA.

Here are some things that are essential for you to look for when choosing a breeder and a puppy. This checklist goes for pedigrees and mongrels alike:

- The mother should live all the time in a normal household setting. If possible try to pick a setting that is similar to your own, especially if you have children.
- Look for signs the mother is actually the mother! This may sound obvious, but some unscrupulous dealers will have any random bitch of the right breed in the house. Look at the interaction between the mother and the puppies. Do they seem at ease and close to each other? Look at the mother's belly. Does she have swollen mammary glands that obviously look like she has recently been feeding young? If the breeder has an excuse why the mother isn't there such as on a walk or at the groomer, either walk away or ask if you can come back at a time when she will be there. It's almost certainly a ploy.

- Watch how the mother and puppies are with you. If the mother is fearful or shy it may mean that the pups have a slight genetic predisposition to the same temperament. It's not a total no-no, but a confident, friendly, happy mother is a good sign. The same goes especially for the puppies. Don't choose a puppy that seems timid, reserved or frightened.
- Ask the breeder about health tests and make sure you know all about the breed before you go. Do not accept any excuses for health test results not being available.
- Ask about preventative healthcare. Make sure you see evidence that the mother is vaccinated regularly. This means the puppies will have some immunity from their mother. Depending on the age of the puppies, they may be vaccinated as well. If they are older than eight weeks they should have had their first vaccination by now. Make sure the mother and puppies have been wormed regularly. Worming is important for puppies and effective products are essential. Do not accept homeopathic vaccines or remedies.
- Ask whether they have a plan for socialisation and habituation. The first few weeks and months of a dog's life are crucial for getting them used to the world at large. I'll be giving you some tips for this in a while, but for now if the breeder doesn't have a plan or doesn't seem to know what these terms mean, walk away.
- Make sure the puppies look well cared for:
    - coat and skin in good condition
    - bright, clear eyes
    - well-nourished, not ribby and thin
    - no signs of fleas
    - no dirty bottoms
    - puppies should be walking or running round with no signs of pain or lameness
    - no laboured breathing or sounds like snoring or grunting
    - no head shaking or smelly ears
- Make sure the breeder is happy for you to come back as many times as is reasonable to make sure you are making the right decision. Be very wary of people trying to get you to hand over money straight away or take the puppy the same day. You should always visit at least three times to make sure everything is consistently good.
- Make sure the breeder is willing to sign the AWF/RSPCA puppy contract. Even if they are an assured breeder with their own contract, ask them to sign yours, too. Not sure what this is? Well, I'm about to tell you ☺

The AWF/RSPCA Puppy Contract

The Animal Welfare Foundation (AWF) is a very little-known charity, but it does fantastic work. I was a trustee for six years, so I know that it uses its money very wisely. The website has great vet and owner information, and the AWF funds a lot of research and education to improve animal welfare. If you have some spare cash or you're looking for a new charity to support, give it a go. When pedigree issues hit the headlines the AWF worked long and hard with the RSPCA to come up with the puppy contract and information pack. There are contracts out there such as the assured breeder one, but they are often heavily weighted in favour of the breeder, not the new owner. We wanted something that would give the new owners some power, redress the balance and give you the potential for comeback if things go wrong.

The puppy information pack that precedes the actual contract is really excellent and gives you all the questions you need to ask the breeder to help ensure, as much as possible, a well-adjusted, healthy puppy. It forms part of the legally binding contract. Even better is that it comes with guidance notes to explain to you (and the breeder if he or she needs them) why those questions are important and what sort of answers you should be looking for. You can find and download the contract easily by Googling it, but the website address should you want it is https://puppy-contract.rspca.org.uk. If you have a breeder that doesn't want to sign it, *walk away*!

Socialisation and Habituation

As I said, this book is about picking your puppy, not how to look after it once you've got it, but I want to touch on something here that's important. It's relevant because these processes must be started by the breeder. The first few weeks of an animal's life are incredibly important for what's called socialisation and habituation. Socialisation is the process by which an animal learns how to identify and interact with its own species, but also with the other species it lives with. Most commonly for dogs this will be humans and cats, but it includes the whole social environment the dog will live in. Failure to socialise a dog properly can result in a dog that is fearful of other dogs or people in general, or has very specific fears such as fear of large dogs, or children, or men with beards! Habituation is the process by which an animal learns to get used to non-threatening things in its environment such as household and neighbourhood sights and sounds, different floor surfaces, wearing a collar and so on.

As the socialisation period starts at three weeks of age you can see that the breeder you choose will have already had a massive influence on this. That's why it's *so* important to be careful about the environment in which your puppy has been raised, and why you should ask your breeder what plan, if any, they have in place for socialisation and habituation. You will be taking over this role and expanding your puppy's experience once it is back home with you, and later when they can go out and about, so it's important you understand what's been done already and what you need to do in the next few weeks.

Ideally, puppies should encounter lots of different sorts of people, including children, elderly people, people with glasses, beards, hats, etc. Bear in mind that when it comes to children, dogs view them quite differently to us. Babies, crawlers, toddlers, under-fives, five- to ten-year-olds and kids over ten appear practically like different species from a dog's point of view. In fact, they appear this bafflingly complex to me too! With this in mind, you need to try and introduce your dog to as many different ages of children as possible. Even more importantly, these need to be happy encounters!

Your dog will also need to be exposed to common household sounds and objects such as the fridge, washing machine, vacuum cleaner, hair-dryers, brooms and so on. This will have to start in the home, but puppies should be carried out and about as soon as it's safe to do so.

Lots of people are confused about how they can manage all this socialisation if the dog isn't allowed out yet. Talk to your vet and make sure you know when its vaccinations will be fully protective, but in the meantime a useful regime to follow is this:

Within seven days of the first vaccine you can start treating your puppy like an adult dog except for not putting it on the ground in a public place – so you can do all their socialisation and habituation except with other dogs. From seven days after the first vaccine you can start to organise play dates like puppy play groups and the like with other puppies or pup-friendly adult dogs (not all adult dogs like pups). The dogs you let your puppy mix with at this stage should either be as vaccinated as yours or fully covered. Just check with your vet about local disease risks.

When you get a new puppy everyone is overwhelmed with how cute it is and it's difficult to keep sight of all the things the dog might encounter later. When I got Badger and Pan we had no kids and we had no friends with kids. We were at that age. The dogs were actually brilliantly socialised and habituated to almost everything because they came everywhere with us, including work, right from a young age. They just didn't encounter kids until, for Badger, it was a bit late. The first child he met properly was a foster boy with behavioural issues of his own, Badger was on a lead, which he virtually never was, and the child practically leapt on his face. In a split second, while we were greeting our friends the boy had forced Badger to the end of his lead and grabbed him for a big close-up face-to-face encounter. I imagine Badger had very rapidly done his entire repertoire of avoidance and communication that to him made it very clear the contact was unwelcome. Ultimately the only option open to him was to nip the offending child. Luckily for all concerned, Badger was a very placid and good-natured dog, so it was just a nip, but it was a scary experience for everyone concerned and a sudden realisation of a big chunk of socialisation we had missed. We won't be making that mistake with the next dog we get. Safe to say, the encounter was not one that endeared Badger to children!

These days there are well-defined and useful lists of suggested things that it's good to consider when you're trying to socialise and habituate your puppy. Many vet practices and behaviourists run puppy classes or groups, which are an opportunity to learn great stuff yourself and get these processes under way for your puppy. One thing that's quite important to remember is that, if you are given a list of things that your puppy should encounter, it's not a speed challenge tick list! If your puppy is in a negative state of mind when they encounter something on your list all you will do is teach them that that thing is bad and the associations can be difficult to undo. This is sensitisation, not habituation. The website ispeakdog.org has some great tips for making sure the first time your dog experiences something it is positive and you don't leave things too late.

A good friend of mine who is a behaviour specialist asked me to make this plea to you: 'For heaven's sake *please* do not snatch the food bowl or chews away from your puppy, always swap for a treat because the former triggers guarding behaviour faster than anything I have ever seen and these issues are lifelong and life-shortening!' Wise words indeed. Try to keep everything as positive as possible and pick your moments wisely. If you're in any doubt, get some good behavioural advice as soon as you can.

On that note, when it comes to behaviour and training 'specialists' be *very* careful. Training and behaviour is totally unregulated in the UK and anyone can call themselves a trainer or behaviourist. For behaviour, make sure whoever you talk to is a member of the Association of Pet Behaviour Counsellors (APBC), or is accredited as a Certified Clinical Animal Behaviourist (CCAB). You can also find qualified veterinary behaviourists (VB) and clinical animal behaviourists (CAB) listed with the Animal Behaviour and Training Council (ABTC).

The days of beating dogs into submission and talking about dominance are well and truly gone. Our understanding of animal behaviour has changed totally since I was a child. Sadly there are many behaviourists and trainers, some very famous ones too unfortunately, who still use negative and aversive methods. This is totally unacceptable and unnecessary. If someone tells you that you need to dominate your dog or use something like a prong collar, don't walk away, *run away*!

Chapter 13

How to Choose a Healthy Kitten

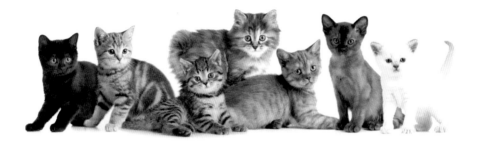

As I have said, some relevant parts of this chapter will be the same as the previous puppy chapter because many people will want either a dog or a cat. If you are reading both chapters out of interest then apologies for the necessary repetition. On the flip side, there are lots of differences too because cats are such fascinating creatures.

As with everything in life, there are no guarantees. There will be those of you out there who have had a moggie with poor health and, of course, there are plenty of pedigree cats that breeze through life with no issues at all. Equally, with the other tips in this chapter they are generalisations; pointers to try and make sure that you avoid the most common pitfalls when it comes to picking a kitten. No one step will guarantee a healthy cat, but if you follow all the steps you've got a much higher chance of having a healthy, well-adjusted pet.

Cats are a little different to dogs in that many people find that they simply acquire a cat without really trying! I've had many clients over the years who have lost a loved, elderly cat and within days another has seemed to sense the void in both the house and the heart and slid in to fill it. Of course, there are also the unplanned litters that still abound in the cat population, so those wonderful moggie kittens are not too difficult to come by.

Some of you will not be quite so lucky and will be actively looking for a cat or kitten. Before we get started on how to go about that, first and foremost, I'd like you to consider adoption. Whether you decide to go for a pedigree or not please remember that there are thousands of cats in adoption centres that need homes. Even if you think you're sure you know what you want, why not just go and have a look? You've got nothing to lose and possibly everything to gain. The good organisations do excellent assessments and help you match a cat to your lifestyle and family circumstances. You never know, you might just fall in love. There's no obligation and you can always walk away. It's also worth considering adopting an older cat. Kittens can be a pain in the bum, no matter how super cute they are. By going for an older cat you're improving the quality of life of that animal immediately and avoiding the pitfalls of litter-training, curtain-climbing and the 4am crawling on to your head because it's time to play!

All I ask is that before you ring someone for the instant gratification kitten online you spend a few hours one afternoon wandering along the aisles of your local adoption centre. Do it for me and if you find something you love let me know on Twitter or Facebook. I'd love to hear about it and, of course, see some photos.

Before you get a Kitten or Cat

So now let's get down to business and the first thing we need to tackle is YOU! One of the biggest causes of abandonment of animals is owners who make the wrong choices. This can be because of breed ill health and unexpected costs, and hopefully I've armed you with the facts in the previous chapters to avoid the worst of those. We'll be looking more clearly at that soon as well.

You need to understand the needs of the cat you are taking on and be *totally honest* with yourself about your situation. This sounds like a blatant plug, and it is, but please consider my *Pet Detective* series to help your research. They are aimed at children, but are great for adults, too. With chapters on each of the five welfare needs and the wild ancestors/relatives to help understand how the animals like to live, they are a useful tool for knowing if any cat is suitable for you. There is also a virtual month for your children or you to complete to give you a taster of what being a cat owner is all about.

The Five Welfare Needs

I mentioned the five welfare needs there and I hope that you are all familiar with them, but surveys every year suggest that many pet owners are still in the dark about these terms. The welfare needs form the basis of the Animal Welfare Act 2006 in England and Wales, the Scottish Animal Health and Welfare Act 2006 and also the Northern Ireland Welfare of Animals Act 2011. The needs are also a brilliant, simple way to approach the care of any animal in the world, captive or wild. By law, in the UK and in many other countries, it is your duty of care to provide for these needs and if you don't you could be prosecuted. Even in places where it isn't the law I believe it is our moral duty to provide for our pets. I've always said that having a pet is a privilege, not a right. Just because you want one doesn't mean you should have one if you can't keep it happy and healthy. The health side of the needs are, in some ways, the easiest to get right. The happiness needs are much more difficult, but *so* important for both the mental wellbeing of your cat and the likelihood of it fitting into your blissful domestic situation!

We'll look at the needs here because it's a good way for you to start to think about your house, life and relationships and how your cat might fit in.

I'll give you a few basic pointers about the needs, but this book is more about picking your pet than looking after it once you've got it. Please listen to your veterinary team and ask them about other respected sources of post-purchase advice. Cats are absolutely fascinating creatures and their behaviour is one of the most misunderstood of all the common pets. The needs are all intertwined, of course, but I see the first three needs listed here as health and the last two as happiness:

1. **The need for a suitable diet and fresh water.** Cats (apart from kittens up to weaning) don't need anything else to drink except water. Fresh water should be available all the time. Lots of cats love running water and you can get fountains for cats that help encourage them to drink. Cats, by nature or in the wild, won't normally drink near their food because if they are eating a dead animal the water supply next to it might be contaminated. Place their water away from their food, or preferably have a few bowls dotted round the house. Cats like wide open bowls so their whiskers don't touch the sides, and they like water bowls full to the brim so they don't have to feel vulnerable by putting their heads right into a bowl.

    When it comes to food there are about a million choices. Which you pick will be your choice and will likely be dictated by things such as your finances and your sources of information, hopefully one of which will be your vet. In general the more expensive the food the better quality and the more controlled/quality-checked it will be. 'Open formula' foods are cheaper and their ingredients may change from batch to batch; for the majority of animals this is fine. Fixed formula foods are more expensive and the ingredients are guaranteed to be the same from batch to batch unless there is an upgrade of some kind. Make sure whatever food you feed is complete and balanced.

    Do not feed raw foods. It presents a significant public health risk, not just to your cat, but to you, your family and the wider population of animals and humans. Home cook food if you want to, but don't feed raw.

    Be aware that kittens need higher energy foods with certain ratios of phosphorous and calcium for healthy growth and joints. They also need specific fatty acids for optimal brain and eye development. I would urge you to feed your kitten a quality, complete kitten food recommended by your vet.

Don't be shy about money. You need to work out how much your cat is going to cost to feed. Cats commonly live to 16 years and more these days, so even the basic costs can be more than you think.

Finally, ask your vet about body condition score, or BCS. This is how to assess if your kitten is the right weight. Obesity is a massive problem now, with many people perceiving fat animals as the right weight. Keep your kitten slim, get into good habits from the word go and they are more likely to stay slim for life, be healthier and live longer. Obesity in cats is very closely linked to bladder issues and especially diabetes. Prevention is always better and easier than cure!

2. **The need for a suitable environment.** For cats this just means your home and garden, but your home might not be suitable for any cat. There are very few cats that are genuinely happy living indoors all the time, so if you live in a flat or don't have a garden then I would seriously question a cat as a suitable pet. Being kept indoors is a major cause of stress, obesity and frustration in cats.

You need to look at the cost of beds, scratch posts and toys and the cost of replacing them. Will your cat be allowed in your bedroom at night? Is your house like a show home and do you want it covered in hair, bodies of wild animals and scratch marks, because if your cat is to be happy your house may well be covered in these things!

3. **The need to be protected from pain, injury and disease.** Veterinary medicine has grown and developed at a similar rate to human medicine. We have the same drugs, surgical equipment, levels of sterility, surgical expertise, medical evaluation and imaging equipment, from a basic X-ray machine to a state-of-the-art MRI scanner. Vets are expensive; that is a fact of modern life. It's not because we are thieving money-grabbers, it's because this stuff costs a lot of money and to ensure the gold standard of care for your pet we have highly trained staff who deserve to be paid for their expertise. People in the UK are used to what appears to be free healthcare for themselves, so we resent paying for care for our animals. As I said, having an animal is a privilege not a right. You need to very carefully consider how much your cat's veterinary care might cost from the most basic vaccination or consultation up to the costs of major surgery should it be needed.

The excellent charity the PDSA produces a yearly report into pet ownership in the UK called the PAW report. It makes for very interesting reading and is readily available online. In the 2017 report a staggering 98% of cat owners underestimated the lifetime costs of owning a cat. The basic minimum cost is around £12,000 and this can go up to £24,000 in some cases, especially where pedigrees are concerned. None of these sums is insignificant, so think carefully about your finances before you take on a kitten.

As for preventing disease, vets recommend vaccination and effective parasite control because it helps keeps your pets safe, alive and comfortable; it's not because we are evil! Please vaccinate your kitten and let it continue on into adulthood. The raging conspiracy theories about vaccination in the human and animal world are dangerous scaremongering and are leading to preventable deaths of animals, children and adults; it's like going back to the Dark Ages. Vaccines save lives. Fact. We all need to be concerned about over-vaccination, but good vets will split vaccines and only give the ones that are necessary. Vaccines are different for different diseases and produce varying lengths of immunity. Some of these need to be given more often than others. Don't listen to the loons saying that animals don't need vaccines. The World Small Animal Veterinary Association (WSAVA) has excellent information on vaccination and it's produced by the leading veterinary experts in the world. If you're concerned about vaccination have a read of the website and vaccine guidelines.

Do not use homeopathic vaccines, or any homeopathic remedies for that matter. They are unscientific, unproven and ineffective.

4. **The need to be kept with or without other animals.** The first of our happiness needs and such an important one. Humans are social animals, even if we don't seem like it sometimes, but cats are not. Humans find it difficult to imagine that a solitary species can be happy alone. There are many cat owners that worry their cat is bored or lonely when they are out so they get another cat to keep them company. Often this is disastrous. Some cats that grow up together stay friends, but many don't. Some cats also seem to cope well with other cats in the house, but many categorically do not.

Cats in the wild and by nature live solitary lives and come together to mate. Where there are feral or semi-feral colonies these are often dictated and maintained by the presence of food and the fundamental point is that cats are free to come and go as they please if they can't cope. Cats in the wild spend vast amounts of time finding food and hunting and they guard their resources fiercely and hate to share. Just because your cat is going to get plenty of love, food and water no matter how many cats you have, it won't stop it seeing the other cat or cats as direct competition for the things it holds most dear. Living with other cats is one of the biggest causes of inappropriate toileting and stress-related problems we see. It is also a major cause of cats leaving to live somewhere else! According to the 2017 PAW report, 42% of cats in the

UK live with another cat and half of those don't get along with one or more of the other cats they live with. Not very happy pets, eh?

5. **The need to behave normally.** Cats do a lot of stuff that humans find annoying, such as killing stuff and scratching the furniture. All animals and humans have behaviours that they have an innate and instinctive need to do. Cats scratch prominent things because they are marking their territory. They don't care how much your sofa cost, it has an important corner on it! They rub on you and try to trip you over because they are marking you as their own. Even if they will never go hungry, many of them have a strong and irresistible urge to chase and catch small mammals and birds even if they don't eat them. You may well find dismembered animals in your house. Don't put bells on your cats; it's very irritating for them and it doesn't stop many of them catching stuff.

The fact is that with any animal you take on you need to know what its normal behaviour is and you have to accept it. You can give your cat things to scratch besides the furniture, but you can't expect your cat not to scratch. If you don't like the sound of the things cats do, don't get one. That same PAW report found that 62% of all cat owners would change something about their cat's behaviour if they could.

Ever wondered why cats always sit on people that hate cats? This is one of my favourite cat facts and is another way that people misunderstand them. Cat lovers love cats. Obviously. They have a tendency to pursue cats, reaching towards them making all sorts of petting sounds. They like to pick cats up and hold them and cuddle them and kiss them. Cats *hate* this. Cats are predators, but they are also prey animals as well. They find being restrained frightening and it cuts off their escape routes. People staring at them and pursuing them makes them vulnerable and threatened. Now picture the cat-hater that arrives in your cat zone. They never look at the cat or go anywhere near it. They positively avoid eye contact in the fear that the devil creature will approach them because they *always do*, which they've never understood. This person is the most attractive, appealing, safe, unthreatening person in the world from a cat's point of view. A happy life with a cat is best achieved on their terms, not yours. The saying, 'Dogs have owners, cats have staff' is absolutely true!

Well, now we've dealt with you we need to start your kitten-picking process. Right from the start let's start to narrow your choices for the good of cat-kind and talk about the elephant in the room straight away; breed health.

Breed Health

I know this whole book so far has been about this, but we need to crystallise that information. Now I know this is going to get me a whole load of abuse from lovers of certain breeds, but I'm not writing this book for them, I'm writing it for people who have an open mind and care deeply about the health of their future beloved pet and want to make the right decision. The title of this book is *Picking a Pedigree?*, but actually I've been a bit sneaky because I don't want you to pick a pedigree! In general you are more likely to get a healthy animal if you pick a moggie. At the moment, until we start breeding for health not looks, all pedigrees by the nature of inbreeding will be more likely to be ill than a moggie. In fact, when it comes to cats I'm going to be pretty categorical and say do not pick a pedigree at all. Cats are a fantastically well-adapted species, largely unspoilt by man, and the pedigrees are unnecessarily poorer deviations from a brilliant baseline.

What comes next is my personal opinion, but I hope I have backed it up with the information in the book. I'm going to list below the breeds that, at this time, I would strongly urge you *not* to buy, either because of extremes of body shape or because of unacceptably high levels of inherited disease. In these breeds, if you do decide to ignore me and go ahead please find out about health testing and do *not* accept a kitten from a breeder that doesn't test and openly share the results. If you ignore me on the extremes of body shape I'll keep my fingers crossed for you! Obviously, I hope that time will change these breeds into less extreme, healthier versions of themselves, so keep an eye out because in another 20 years this list might be very different. I hope it will be non-existent, but I've been hoping that for the last 20 years! I must for balance point out that there are, of course, some individuals of these breeds that have had no health issues at all. I'm steering you away from these breeds because I believe that they are the worst affected on the whole, so if you avoid them you are already ahead of the game when it comes to your chances of a healthy specimen.

As I said, if you stick to the moggies you won't go far wrong, but there are extremes in cats too so I've listed the worst affected. In different countries there are many various crosses and other versions of some of these too, so remember the earlier chapters and watch out for the extremes. Bear in mind that, although conformational problems are the same almost everywhere, the inherited diseases do vary a little from country to country. Make sure you find out about the gene pools where you live.

There are many varieties of fold cats, hairless cats and tail-less cats springing up in different countries. All of these should be avoided for the reasons we have listed for the most well-known breeds.

Breeds to avoid	Reason
Exotic shorthair	Brachycephalic
Manx	Inherited disease
Munchkin	Extremes
Persian	Brachycephalic and inherited disease
Siamese	Extremes and inherited disease
Scottish fold	Inherited disease
Sphynx	Extremes

It's worth pointing out here that there are some breeders doing their utmost to breed for older versions of some of these breeds regardless of what wins shows. Some of the old-style Persian breeders, for example, have made a point of maintaining the less extreme lines and have totally avoided the horrible concave faces and extremely long coats. Some of these old-style cats really do resemble those much more moderate Persians of the early 1900s and, of course, the best breeders will health test, too (see Figures 13.1 to 13.4). More of that in the next chapter.

Breed and Moggie Characteristics

As we said, cats like life on their own terms. Many people love cats because they are independent and don't have the clingy needs of some dogs. Some people who get cats make the mistake of thinking they can guarantee a lap cat and end up sorely disappointed when theirs seems to view them as an unwelcome smell!

Obviously, for most cat owners their temperament is important. Whether your cat likes sitting with you may not be important, but no one wants a cat that savages you and your family every time you walk into the room.

Some cats are friendlier than others and some of this will be altered by their early experiences, but some of it will be genetic. Our good old moggies are just cats, so you won't know their make-up and often the father will be totally unknown, but there are still ways you can get an inkling of what their personality will be if you meet them and their mum when the kittens are very young. We'll be looking at that in a minute.

As for the known breeds, some will have reputations for having certain tendencies, just the same as dog breeds differ. Some people see Siamese and Burmese as more social cats, so they may be best avoided if you're out all day. It's also really important to consider breed health with respect to behaviour. Many people describe Persians as placid, but some of this will be because some of them have such trouble breathing that they don't do much else. Many Persians

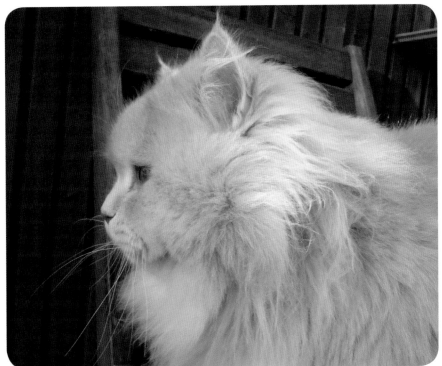

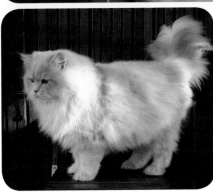

Figures 13.1, 13.2: Egerton Geovarni – a beautiful old-style Persian. Notice his nose position ... (Photo: www.klassiskperserkat.dk)

also hate being groomed and this can lead to behavioural conflict with their owners. The hairless cats get labelled as social, but it could be simply because they are so dependent on their owners for care and are often kept indoors to keep warm. Classically, a lot of vets now see Bengal cats and similar breeds for marked behavioural problems, but much of this could be because they are such striking and expensive cats that many are kept indoors. As I have said, this can cause huge stress and frustration in cats.

Remember, just because a breed has a tendency to be a certain way it's no guarantee and their early experiences can still change them a lot.

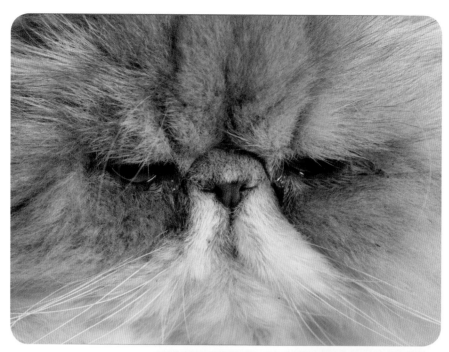

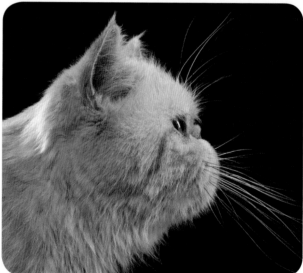

Figures 13.3, 13.4: ...compared to a modern Persian. (Photo: Adobe Stock)

Finding a Kitten and What to Look for

As I said at the beginning of this chapter, quite often your cat will find you. Most vets I know end up with cats because they are the waifs and strays, unwanted, abandoned or neglected, that end up at the surgery. Certainly, all of my cats have come along like that! You may hear of someone in your neighbourhood with a litter of accidental kittens or see a notice in the supermarket. Adoption centres are an excellent place to start looking if you want to actively find a cat. They often have kittens, or you may also find a young cat that you fall in love with. Good adoption organisations will have tried to make sure that kittens are well social-ised and habituated where possible. They will also have excellent advice for you on litter training, vaccinations and so on. Do not buy a kitten from a pet shop; you will never know what environment they were born and raised in and never see the mother.

If you go to a breeder, whether they are moggies or pedigrees, there are certain things you should look for in both the cats and the breeders. The bottom line is this; if there is *anything* that makes you feel ill at ease, you *walk away*. Even if you feel sorry for a little rag-scrag kitten, do not take it on; you will simply be funding a poor breeder and may well be taking on a lifetime of vets' bills and a sickly animal.

You may have an idea about what colour of cat you'd prefer or the length of its coat, but temperament and health are so important for a family pet, so make them your priority.

Socialisation and Habituation

As I said, this book is about picking your kitten not how to look after it once you've got it, but this is very important because these processes must be started by the breeder. The first few weeks of an animal's life are incredibly important for what's called socialisation and habituation. Socialisation is the process by which an animal learns how to identify and interact with its own species, but also with the other species it lives with. Most commonly for cats this will be humans, other cats (remember this is not always a good thing) and dogs, but it includes the whole social environment the cat will live in. Habituation is the process by which an animal learns to get used to non-threatening things in its environment and be comfortable with them.

Three to seven weeks of age is a crucial part of this, so you can see that the breeder you choose will have already had a massive influence. That's why it's *so* important to be careful about the environment in which your kitten has been raised and ask your breeder what plan, if any, they have in place for socialisation and habituation. You will be taking over this role and expanding your kitten's experience once it moves to your house and goes out and about, so it's important you understand what's been done already and what you need to do in the next few weeks.

Ideally, kittens should encounter, and be gently handled by, lots of different sorts of people. If your kitten is not used to being handled by people they may only ever just about tolerate human contact, but may not enjoy it. Your kitten will also need to be habituated to familiar things in the house, such as the noise of the vacuum and so on. This also needs to be done in the right way to avoid simply making the kittens scared instead of calm.

This process will have to start in the breeder's home. Ideally, try to find a kitten that's been raised in a similar situation to your house, especially if you have a dog or children. Many cats live really well with dogs and can be much happier with a dog than another cat. That said, you have to be sure your dog feels the same way!

Signs of Health and What to Ask

Make sure you ask the breeder what their vaccination schedule is and what vaccines, if any, the kitten has had. Depending on their age, they may not have had any yet, but ask for evidence that the mother (and father if known) are vaccinated regularly. Also ask about worming. Worming is very important around pregnancy, lactation and early life. Ask what products have been used and check with your vet whether they are effective.

As I said, try to get an idea of the temperament of the mother. Does she seem relaxed and comfortable with humans? Bear in mind that if she is a new mum or the kittens are very small she may be protective of them. Hopefully the breeder will have been handling the kittens from birth, so the mum should be used to that, too. Ask if you can handle the kittens. This way you can see if they are relaxed with you. Try to see all of them to see how they are.

Look for a clean environment. Of course, there may be a little bit of poo and wee, but if the house seems messy and dirty or there are cats everywhere be wary. Good hygiene is very important for the health of young animals. In places that breed a lot of animals it is easy for cats to have chronic issues, such as infectious diseases including chlamydia. It's really important to try and see if all the cats are in good health. Don't accept a kitten that has *any* signs that it is not 100% fit and healthy. Here's what to look for:

- Coat and skin in good condition, make sure no matts or bald patches, sores or scabs. Look for fleas or flea dirt in the coat.
- Bright, clear eyes. Runny eyes are a common sign of poor health and infectious disease. Do not be fobbed off with stories or any excuses if you see this. Eyes should be open, wide and clear. If the kittens or cats have red eyes, swollen eyes or seem to be squinting, walk away.
- Well-nourished, not ribby and thin. This might be difficult to tell depending on the coat length, so make sure you feel them.

- No dirty bottoms. Cats are fastidiously clean, so dirty bottoms won't be a good sign.
- Kittens, depending on their age, should be moving around with no signs of pain or lameness. They should also be active. If one or more of them seems to be sleeping every time you visit then be very wary; this could be a sign of general ill-health or congenital disease.
- No laboured breathing or sounds like snoring or grunting. Cats breathe almost exclusively through their noses and only mouth breathe if they are ill or very distressed. Noses should be clear from mucus and crusts.
- No head shaking or smelly, dirty ears.

Make sure the breeder is happy for you to come back as many times as is reasonable to make sure you are making the right decision. Be very wary of people trying to get you to hand over money straight away or take the kitten the same day. You should always visit at least three times before you take a kitten to make sure that what you are seeing is consistently good.

If you're getting a pedigree make sure you have found out about the possible health problems within that breed. If there are health tests available it is essential you pick a breeder that does these tests and is open and happy to share the results. There is no excuse not to, so don't be fooled with reasons why. Try to avoid breeders advertising multiple breeds or that have large breeding colonies. These are less likely to have well-adjusted animals simply because of the numbers of kittens being produced.

Hopefully I've given you a good grounding in what to look out for and what to avoid. For the ongoing care of your kitten or cat if you want excellent information of every aspect of cat health, welfare and care go to the International Cat Care website. It is a fantastic charity and welfare organisation and its advice is absolutely up to date and spot on.

We've mentioned health testing several times throughout the book, so now we are nearing the end of our little journey through cats and dogs it's time to look at what could, and really *should,* be done about health.

Chapter 14

Health – What Can and Should be Done

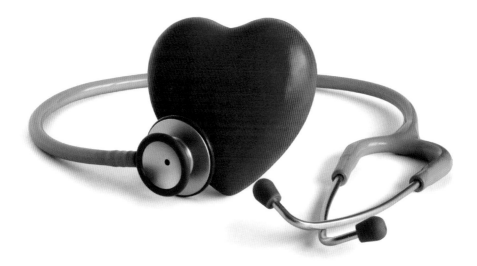

NOW WE'VE LOOKED AT THE GENERAL THINGS YOU CAN DO TO CHOOSE a puppy or kitten most likely to be happy as well as healthy I think it's time to look more closely at what we can all do about health. There are lots of stakeholders when it comes to our pets' health and if we all start working harder and together hopefully we can make some really positive changes in the near future.

The number of tests for inherited disease is enormous and is evolving all the time, so I won't begin to try to cover all of them here. Knowing that some of these tests have been around in the UK since the mid-1970s should make us ask ourselves why pedigree health seems to be much the same or possibly even worse when so many tests are available to breeders to improve the health of their offspring. The horrible answer to this is because so many breeders don't do the tests and some breeders do the tests and breed from animals regardless of poor results.

One of the longest-running schemes is the hip dysplasia scheme. As we said in the inherited disease chapter, this condition is very common in certain breeds, two of the most well-known being the Labrador and the German shepherd dog. The British Veterinary Association (BVA) and the KC run the scheme and the results are readily available. The hip scheme is available for any dog and the rolling 15-year averages are shown for dozens of breeds.

The test involves having an X-ray taken of the hips, which is then examined by orthopaedic experts. They look at a number of factors and give each hip a score from 0–53, producing a total score out of 106. Perfect hips are a 0; the higher the score, the worse the hips. A breed average is produced and the advice, quite rightly, is not to breed from any animal that doesn't have a score *well below* the breed average. Over time this should result in only dogs with good hips being bred from.

At the time of writing the breed average for the German shepherd over the last 15 years is 11 and over the last five years it's also 11. The Labrador is nine and nine. This means that in two of the breeds most affected by this crippling disease the hips have not improved in recent years. One of the issues with the data is that the averages are probably not truly representative of the breed as a whole. If someone has an X-ray taken and their own vet at the time can see that the hips are poor it is not uncommon for the breeder to simply choose not to submit the X-ray. This saves them the cost of the assessment when they already know the answer is poor. This means that there is a likelihood that some poor hips are not being submitted and are therefore not being included, giving the breed an apparently better average than it has. So it would help if it was compulsory for breeders and vets to submit any X-rays taken with the intention of being used for the scheme. This would enable much more accurate data to be collected.

Of course, by far and away the most enormous problem with the scheme, and many of the others, is that they are not compulsory themselves! I have repeatedly asked the KC why it does not make certain health schemes mandatory for animals to be registered. If a breeder phones the KC to register a litter of Labrador puppies and is denied because the parents were not hip scored and proven to have hips below the average, that breeder would soon be adhering to best practice, not breeding or producing unregistered litters that would be worth less or less likely to sell.

As always it is the unsuspecting owners as well as the animals that suffer the heartbreak and the fall-out from this. When I worked in Cheltenham we had a lovely Labrador puppy that we saw from the age of its first vaccination. Her owner was keen to breed from her and we had recommended hip scoring. He didn't know anything about it so we gave him all the information and shortly after her first birthday we booked her in to have her X-ray taken as per the regulations. By horrible coincidence, about a week before the X-ray she went lame on her back leg. When we took the X-ray we could see her hips were awful, the pain already becoming apparent. We submitted the X-rays because, as I said, it's important for data collection. Her score was 96 (see Figures 14.1 and 14.2). Absolutely appalling.

Her owner was livid and became very angry with us, not through malice, simply because he was venting his frustration. He raved around the consulting room,

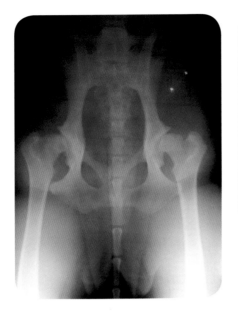

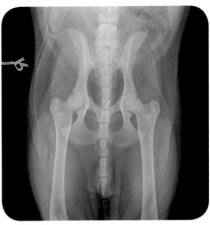

Figure 14.1 (left): Labrador hips with a score of 96.

Figure 14.2 (above): Normal hips sit snugly in their sockets. (Photo: Andy Moores)

fuming. He had contacted her breeder and been told, inevitably, that her parents were not tested. How could this be possible he asked? How could she have been registered if this test was so important for the breed and hadn't been done? I had no answer for him because I'd been wondering the same thing for a decade by then. A young dog was crippled for life because of a breeder who was at best ignorant and at worst uncaring and selfish. It was something that could have been stopped rapidly with compulsory health testing.

So what of the German shepherd? German shepherds, as we said, have changed radically in the show ring in recent years. Their sloping backs and bizarre gait make them waddle like ducks and bunny hop when they run, almost looking unable to stand unaided in some cases. Their hip scores are unchanged in the last 15 years. In 2016 at Crufts the winner of best of breed for the German shepherd caused a public outcry because she appeared so crippled when she was paraded round the ring. The breeder defended the dog and said that she had been hip scored, implying she had good hips. When I visited the website I found her score was 13. The BVA recommends that dogs should not be bred from unless their hip score is well below the breed average. The breed median is 11; 13 is not well below it!

The breeder says on its site, 'All our parents are hip and elbow scored with results within the breed average', which it states is below 20 for hips. The breeder obviously has a different interpretation of the BVA statistics to me. The website proudly goes on to say what a good mother the bitch was. She has already been bred from, one of her offspring having a hip score of 16. Worse than her mother, but going by the breeder's rather lenient take on the breed average obviously still fine!

In another twist that leaves me not sure whether to laugh or cry, after the uproar in 2016, the KC changed the GSD breed standard to include 'additional wording to emphasise the importance of the dogs being capable of standing comfortably and calmly, freely and unsupported in any way'. Someone has actually taken the time to write down that it's preferable if a dog, that in the wild is one of the most successful types of species on the planet, should be able to stand unaided! It is a statement almost as blindingly obvious as the bulldog standard declaring 'signs of respiratory distress highly undesirable'! Let us not forget that at the outset these animals were working dogs similar to Border collies. How is it possible that the show world has been allowed to get away with crippling a dog that should be capable of running for hours every day? Once more, if you look back at photographs of German shepherds from decades ago they have high rumps like wolves and coyotes, not backs that slope off into a diseased abyss (see Figures 14.3 and 14.4).

There are some people who criticise the hip dysplasia scheme even though many countries use this method of X-ray evaluation. There is a different scheme being used in some areas now called the PennHIP scheme, which is also based on an X-ray evaluation, but the hind legs and hips are put into a different position. The proponents of this scheme feel that it is less likely to accidentally show fairly poor hips in a good light, which they feel is possible with the traditional view used. Time and further evidence gathering will undoubtedly tell. Perhaps we will end up with

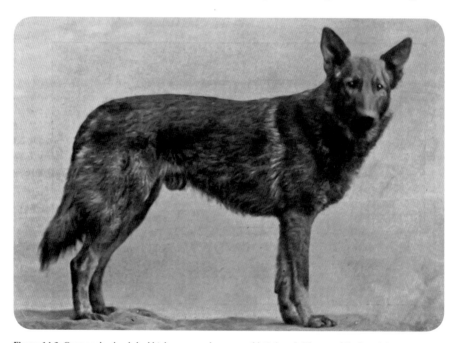

Figure 14.3: German shepherds had high rumps and were an athletic breed. (Photo: public domain)

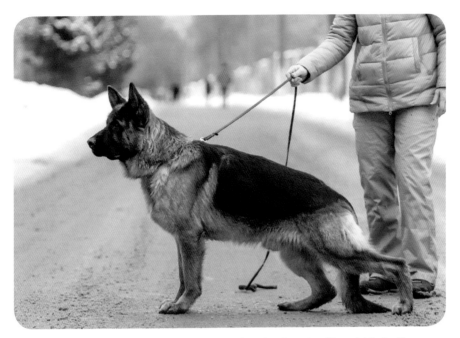

Figure 14.4: Some modern dogs are crippled by this newly desired conformation. (Photo: Adobe Stock)

a combination of the two for absolute clarity. To my mind, even if the current test has some shortcomings, it certainly does identify many bad hips and the more we can eliminate these individuals from the breeding schemes the better.

The fact is that show-winners are highly sought after for breeding. Unhealthy specimens, especially males, can go on to produce multitudes of offspring all carrying their defective genes or conformation, what we call a genetic bottleneck. Surely we should expect dogs winning any shows of this type to be the absolute pinnacle of good health, let alone the winners of the biggest shows on earth? In 2011 vet checks were introduced at Crufts and other championship shows. These checks are only for what the KC calls category three breeds on its breed watch list. The KC breed watch list scores all breeds between one and three. Breeds in category one have no points of concern, category two some points of concern and category three are 'breeds where some dogs have visible conditions or exaggerations that can cause pain or discomfort'.

The dogs don't have to pass a vet check to enter the show in the first place, but if they win best of breed they must have a check before being allowed to have the title confirmed and progress into the group competition. Now there are a few things to bear in mind with this. These vet checks are looking for visible signs of things that may cause pain, discomfort or problems with walking and moving. Firstly, these checks are clearly not working if a shepherd such as the one in 2016 can both win

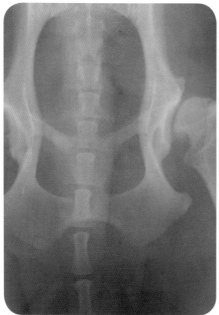

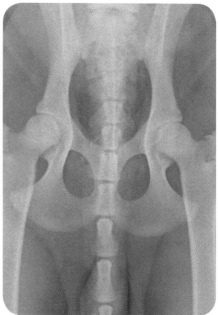

Figure 14.5: Severe hip dysplasia in a GSD ...

Figure 14.6: ... compared to those lovely normal hips we saw before. (Photo: Andy Moores)

best of breed *and* progress to the group competition in the biggest dog show in the world, and secondly the breed watch list is far from ideal.

The Cavalier spaniel we've talked so much about already is classed as category one – no points of concern. Erm ... Really? Now I'm assuming and hoping that the vet checks include listening to the chest and seeing as the prevalence of heart disease in the breed is totally unacceptably high you'd think they'd be in a different category and get an occasional once over before being crowned a super breeding specimen!

Talking about cavalier hearts, what can breeders do about MVD? In the late 1990s a group of specialist cardiologists from around the world came up with a breeding protocol that they felt could be used to try and eliminate or reduce MVD in Cavaliers. The protocol states that dogs should not be bred from before the age of two and a half years and, of course, should be heart clear (i.e. no murmur audible) and they should have parents that are heart clear at the age of five years. In fact, the specialists felt that no Cavaliers should be bred from before the age of five years, but reduced it to two and a half years in an attempt to find an acceptable compromise. You would think that with almost every dog being afflicted with this disease by the age of ten and almost half of them dying of this disease that breeders would have immediately welcomed this protocol and started using it.

Guess again. Back at Crufts, this time in 2017, the best of breed, I repeat, *best* of breed, cavalier at Crufts had literally just turned two and a half. According to the KC website, he had already sired seven litters, 23 puppies in the UK, the first time being just after his first birthday. The second litter he sired was born to the bitch belonging to the breed club's own health representative. If the breed club's *own health representative* doesn't follow the protocol what hope is there for the people looking to buy these puppies?

After this travesty the people at Cavaliers Are Special decided to do a bit of digging to see if this was indeed an exception to the rule. A blog they wrote on their research says this:

> This made us wonder: was this year's Crufts best of breed winner just a very high-profile exception to the rule, and are top show breeders and breed club officials setting a good example for others to follow. Cavaliers Are Special decided to do some research into underage matings – those with one or both parents under the age of two and a half.
>
> The Cavalier Club awards trophies based on points won during the year. We analysed the age at which the top Cavaliers in three categories were bred from 2012 to 2016 inclusive (114 Cavaliers). The three trophies were for the Cavalier scoring the most individual points, best stud dog and best brood bitch. The latter two categories are based on points scored by their progeny.
>
> Of the 755 litters bred by these Cavaliers in the five years we examined, 30% had one or both parents under two and a half years old.
>
> We also looked at which of these Cavaliers were owned by past and present Cavalier Club committee members and office holders, and past and present regional and national puppy coordinators – referred to as the Club Committee/Puppy Coordinator group. Of the 345 litters bred by this group, 39% had one or both parents under two and a half years old. In contrast, non-compliance with breeding guidelines with breeders outside of this group was just 23%.

It seems pretty clear that the people who could and really should be affecting change are not overly keen on safeguarding their own dogs' health, let alone that of the entire breed. In fact, studies suggest that only about 4% of breeders in the UK follow the protocol.

As we said in a previous chapter, in the UK the life expectancy of these dogs has gone *down* in recent years. In contrast the Danish KC and CKCS breed club has had mandatory heart testing since 2002. Its protocol uses both auscultation and ultrasound. This extract from the website cavalierhealth.org explains it:

> The protocol is a modification of the standard MVD protocol. Currently, the male and female breeding dogs first must be examined by auscultation and echocardiograph at the age of 18 months, or later by veterinarians approved by the Danish Kennel Club. If a dog is found to be clear of MVD, it is issued a breeding certificate which is valid until the dog reaches the age of four years and a month. If the dog is to be bred after that age, it must be re-examined, found clear of MVD, and receive another certificate, which, for females, is valid for life. For males, the second certificate is valid until age six years and a month. If the male is to be bred after that age, he must be examined and certified a third time.

The club has since found that between 2002 and 2011 there has been a massive 71% reduction in the risk of MVD. In the same time, dogs that did not follow the protocol had no reduction in heart disease. This is pretty difficult to argue with when it comes to the need for such major health tests to be mandatory and effective.

Besides the hip dysplasia scheme, the KC and BVA also run schemes for elbow dysplasia, and an eye scheme that checks for many inherited eye conditions and, more recently, as I mentioned in the Teacups and Giants chapter, the CM/SM scheme for syringomyelia.

When we do welfare assessments, one way to look at things such as health issues is how common the disease is, how much suffering it causes and how long that suffering lasts. For example, lifelong respiratory compromise in more than half of brachycephalics would rate pretty highly for welfare impact, while a small percentage of a hypothetical breed dropping dead of a heart attack at the age of 16 might be of less concern.

When you talk to the owners of dogs with CM/SM it is clear what unbearable suffering the moderate to severe cases of this cause, and it's lifelong. Sometimes that will be a greatly shortened life because it's not uncommon for dogs to be euthanased due to uncontrollable pain. With the prevalence of this disease being so high, especially in clinically silent dogs, it seems to me it's imperative that breeders are compelled to act. If the dogs are not screened how can we know if the silent ones are passing on the defect or not?

The scheme started in 2012 and involves MRI imaging of the dog's skull, brain and the top of the spinal cord. The dogs are then given a grade of 0, 1 or 2 for both CM and SM. These are then broken down into ages with the recommendation that they are scanned at around one, three and five years of age. The numbers taking the scheme up were extremely low, with some breeders actively boycotting the scheme for reasons known only to themselves. Some say it's too expensive. To get an MRI done three times could cost up to £500 a time. When I scanned the online ads for cavalier puppies they range in price from £600 to £1,500 each. It seems like the costs would soon be covered …

As of July 2017, on the official BVA/KC scheme 413 CKCS have been scanned. In *five* years. In that same time more than *twenty thousand* CKCS puppies have been registered by the KC. In an effort to boost numbers being graded the KC actually did a good thing in 2015 and set aside a whopping £30,000 for people who wanted older scans to be looked at. At the time of writing just 19 historical scans have been graded. Wow, those breeders sure do care.

Over my time as a vet I have heard many people tell me that breeders love their animals and it's not all about the money. Let me say unequivocally that I know this is true for some. I have encountered and spoken to breeders who have been categorically dedicated to the health of their animals and have done everything in their power to ensure healthy offspring. *But* my experience, and the experience of countless other vets, and the lack of health testing even among the breed clubs and show winners leads me to believe that breeders like this are sadly in the minority.

Besides these tests there are many other genetic tests available for different breeds with the Animal Health Trust (AHT) among others offering dozens of tests for dogs and cats alike. The AHT is constantly doing research into inherited diseases and good breeders should be aware of their breed's potential problems, aware of what tests are available and should be willing to be honest about whether the tests have been done *and* open about the results. If you visit the AHT website, it has a full list by breed and what they can be tested for. It's an excellent website for information.

It's important to note here that many animal diseases are investigated and have extensive genetic and medical research if they are also applicable diseases for humans. This means that there may be tests available for diseases that are actually pretty rare in a breed and of little significance. I realise this doesn't help you much as a consumer, but just be aware of it. If a breeder hasn't done every test possible for a breed don't write them off, but make sure you understand what tests are available and ask which ones have been done, and most importantly why. Alarm bells should definitely ring if they don't even seem to know what, if any, tests are available for the breed.

Let's go back to the category three breeds and the epitome of poor breed health – the brachys. Bulldogs, pugs and Pekes are on the category three list at this time, French bulldogs, for some reason, are not. There are huge amounts of research being done into BOAS and the respiratory problems faced by these breeds. I also think it's important to remember their many other issues, such as eye, dental, spinal and skin disease and difficulties giving birth as well, but of course, whether a dog can breathe and cool itself effectively trumps everything.

There are many universities all over the world looking at these things and various approaches to trying to objectively measure the problem. The study at Cambridge, which we mentioned in the graphics back in Chapter 3, has used a measure of respiratory flow called whole body barometric plethysmography or, thankfully, WBBP for short! This involves the dogs being placed in a large, transparent, sealed box with equipment attached to measure the changes in the air movement and pressure inside the box as the dogs breathe. It's totally non-invasive and the group has looked at various brachy breeds and compared the breathing patterns to non-brachy animals of a similar size of various breeds and cross-breeds.

Alongside the WBBP, in these studies other things were examined to try to give the dogs overall grades of BOAS. The animals are examined before and after an exercise tolerance test and an extensive history taken, including temperature, body condition (whether the animal is overweight) and also, interestingly, the owner's perception of whether the dog has any problems with its breathing. Each dog is graded from 0 to 3, where 0 is clear of BOAS, 1 is slightly affected but not showing clinical signs, and 2–3 are increasingly severe with grade 3 having life-threatening levels of obstruction. The results from these studies are, as we saw, tragic.

All the non-brachy dogs across the board are grade 0. They are clinically free of obstructive airway disease, as you may imagine they would be. Animals are, after all, ideally capable of breathing normally. Around 50% of bulldogs, 58% of French bulldogs and a whopping 64% of pugs were grade 2–3. This means that these animals are either in need of intervention and have signs of respiratory distress, or in the case of grade 3s may have the need for immediate surgical intervention for life-threatening problems. This is something we need to address right now, not by trying to gradually breed for slightly different conformation over the next 20 generations.

Scarily, as we said, almost 60% of owners of these affected animals had not noticed any respiratory issues. This goes back to the accepted 'norm' that pugs and such dogs snore and pant a lot. It's *not normal*. This lack of comprehension means many animals are not presented for intervention until the disease has progressed and the outcome likely to be poorer.

One study also found that bulldogs and pugs were much more likely to be obese than normal animals, with 62% of pugs being deemed clinically obese. If you cast your mind back to their breed standard, which says they should never be lean or leggy, maybe the owners can be forgiven for thinking that that is what a pug is 'supposed' to look like. Sadly, the effects of obesity on animals or humans when it comes to exercise tolerance and heat control are very well-known. Inflict those added stresses on an animal with a compromised airway and you have got a pretty dreadful life.

Exercise tests seem a good functional test we should be doing for all brachy animals. The test required for the studies I've just mentioned involved the dogs being trotted for a period of three minutes, other countries choose different things. Germany and Finland have tests that involve the dogs having to cover a distance of 1,000m in a certain time. Some owners and breeders have complained that the tests are too strenuous, which speaks volumes in itself. If any of my dogs struggled to trot for three minutes or walk a kilometre in ten minutes I would have serious concerns about their health!

One of the fundamental things that comes up time and again with many of our most diseased breeds is that their gene pools are already so small. In the brachy studies it seems that less than 10% of pugs and around 10% of Frenchies are grade 0 for BOAS. Even if we're lenient and let the grade 1s breed, you're still reducing the gene pool by half or more. Goodness knows what we'd end up with then. Outcrossing or banning the breeds are rapidly becoming the only acceptable solutions; or at least let's see function tests being made mandatory for breeding status or show entry at any level.

So what else could be done besides health tests? Vets, law-makers, the KC and cat fancy associations and insurance companies could all play a role, I believe.

Laws

In 2016 two breeders of Persian cats in Switzerland were prosecuted under the country's 'Qualzucht' laws. This translates as 'torture breeding', which is a necessarily powerful name I think. Many of our worst affected breeds you could argue are born to suffer. They have a life of torture inflicted on them by the body shapes and genes we've bred into them. Producing animals with a high likelihood of suffering should, of course, be against the law, just the same as beating an animal is. If you inflict pain and suffering through any means you should be held responsible. Our current laws don't apply to embryos, but surely when a mating is so likely to cause disease as found in some of our most unhealthy cats and dogs, those setting out to do that should be prosecuted.

The European Convention for the Protection of Pet Animals was created in 1987 and many countries have signed and ratified it. One section tackles extremes of conformation and could be used to prosecute the worst offenders. The UK neither signed nor ratified it, according to one newspaper article because of 'lobbying by some in the pedigree dog breeding world who believed that their activities might be restricted by the elements of Qualzucht that the Convention introduced'. Worrying indeed. When breeders are worried they might be accused of torture breeding they know something is badly wrong.

Everyone hates the word 'ban', but throughout history we have banned many, many things that have come to be seen as unacceptable. Slavery, smoking in public, drink-driving, text-driving, capital punishment, bear-baiting, cock fighting and, of course, the list goes on. Crimes of very varying importance depending on your views, I'm sure. The disastrous Dangerous Dogs Acts makes the mere mention of banning breeds almost impossible, but I believe we have reached a critical threshold of disease for some of these breeds. Laws should be introduced that make health testing, outcrossing and anything else deemed necessary for health and welfare mandatory. If that means some breeds disappear then so be it. We made them, we can say goodbye to them, too. Back to the drawing board of pet 'design'.

The fact is that the UK puts itself forward as a huge leader in animal welfare, but we are laughably behind many other countries. We could have legislation to make registration of all or at least some pets compulsory. This would make tracking pet numbers much easier at the very least. Some countries have laws that say owners must produce proof of knowledge about a certain animal before they can have one. What a great idea! How can we prosecute people for making stupid choices if we don't make sure they are educated first? It would be like convicting someone of dangerous driving without insisting on a driving test. Prospective owners could either be expected to pass an exam about the pet they want or prove that they have 'grandfather knowledge'.

It seems sensible too, by law, to insist that anyone wanting to breed a dog or cat at least should be licensed and inspected regularly. There must be more we can do globally to crack down on puppy farms. Each breeder should have a registration number that is applied to every puppy advertised to allow transparency. The Dog Breeding Reform Group is a really excellent organisation that is dedicated to improving these issues and it has devised a very comprehensive standard for dog breeding, which you can find on its website. This should be made the gold standard for breeding by law.

The trading standards rules should be changed to make it illegal to use the worst affected animals in any advertising or marketing. This would be an agreed and ever-evolving list agreed by veterinary experts. The use of quirky, diseased animals in advertising is disgusting and massively drives the continued demand for these animals.

It would also be good to see legislation and those making the laws empowering vets more and actually listening to veterinary associations. Too often when it comes to animal welfare matters it seems to be the wealthy, vocal, interested minority that is listened to over and above the very people extensively trained to understand the subject better than anyone.

During the editing of this book it's come to light that there may well be some new laws coming in the UK at the end of 2018. These could include much stricter rules about puppy sales and breeder licensing but also, hugely importantly, laws that may include future offspring like the torture breeding laws. I truly hope so.

I believe that we should have an independent, expert veterinary panel appointed by WSAVA to review every breed standard in the world. These experts should identify every sentence that translates as selection for genetic disease, extremes of conformation and physical abnormalities compared to natural canids and felids and these standards should be outlawed and changed or abolished immediately. The selection *for* any physical or genetic abnormality is morally indefensible.

The KC and Breed Clubs

I feel as if I've been banging my head on this wall for long enough now. The KC could make huge differences to health and welfare, but it has failed to do so adequately. Yes, it has done some positive things in the last decade, but it could do so much more. It repeatedly says it feels it's best to leave testing to breeders' discretion, but this is categorically failing to make a difference. Many other countries and their breed clubs and KCs have introduced mandatory tests for various conditions and function tests, yet ours so far refuses to do so. The latest word is that the KC are finally going to introduce a heart scheme based on the Danish one and it will be mandatory for assured breeders. This is great news and I hope they will soon widen the net and make it necessary for every cavalier breeder wanting to register a puppy with them, not just the assured breeders.

The KC's frequently stated reason is that it is concerned that breeders would leave the group and go underground. It fears that this would lead to more problems with health and welfare. My reply to this has always been this: The KC heralds itself as the foremost organisation that cares about the health and welfare of all dogs. If it loses poor breeders by insisting on health and function tests then so be it. The remaining breeders become the best of the best. The KC talks about its Assured Breeder Scheme. Why not insist that every breeder meets these requirements? Why shouldn't we expect that? How better to avoid the occasional accidental, unplanned litters being registered? The club has a commitment, it says of the scheme, to stamp out puppy farms, but yet it must be registering puppies from large-scale producers you could arguably call farms. Stamp them out? Make every KC breeder an assured breeder, and make the scheme better.

The Kennel Club might lose numbers to start with, but pretty soon breeding standards and health would be improving incredibly quickly. The KC registration could start to be a sign of good things, rather than a profit-making body potentially shielding breeders with poor practices.

The vet checks are not working. Animals should have to pass vet checks prior to entry into any championship show, let alone Crufts. All animals should be checked, not just category three. It's totally ridiculous that animals are being allowed to reach Crufts when they can't walk normally or unaided, or breathe normally, or have overt signs of disease. How can French bulldogs not be examined for signs of respiratory distress when they are the second worst-affected breed? The vets should be appointed by the likes of the BVA or BSAVA to ensure they are completely independent and not answerable to breeders, showers or the KC.

Show winners should be the healthiest dogs you can find. At 2017 Crufts, 'brachy day', there were reports in the media of the heating being switched off in the hall with the brachys in it. Health concerns should never be covered up and animals allowed to suffer. Breed clubs should be following and widely promoting recommended protocols. The current state of affairs is tragically poor.

The KC could introduce a rule that any breed that reaches number three on the watch list is not allowed to be shown until the clubs prove that they have tackled the issues and notably improved health. I'd rather this was for any breed when those such as the CKCS are not even considered to have issues, but I'd take the number threes as a good place to start. It would soon motivate breed clubs to keep health as a priority for fear of getting knocked off the allowed-to-show list.

Insurance Companies

Insurance companies need to start being more strict in a couple of areas. One is that, as already happens in some countries, they should refuse to pay for corrective surgery, such as BOAS surgery, and operations including spinal surgery in dachshunds. This sounds very harsh for the individuals first impacted, but breed disease and the correction of it is increasingly raising premiums and putting pressure on insurance companies and other owners. We need to deter people from buying the worst-affected breeds and finances are a good starting point. We should be encouraging owners to choose healthy animals rather than faddy, popular, diseased ones.

Insurance companies need to make it clear to vets that when a new puppy or kitten is examined for signs of existing disease we need to be including things that are 'normal for the breed', but would actually be considered abnormal, diseased or deformed in a mongrel or moggie. Examples would be any BOAS-related things such as stenotic nostrils, dental malocclusion, chondrodystrophy, diamond eye and so on. This would again start to make owners aware of the likely issues the animals might have later in life and stop abnormalities and disease being seen as normal.

Vets

We need to stop seeing these things as normal, too. We are becoming as habituated to it as everyone else. It's *not normal*. We need to start being more direct with both owners and breeders. We are constantly fighting a losing battle because we always see the animals after acquisition. Of course, it is virtually never the new owner's fault they have picked an unhealthy breed, so we try to be kind and diplomatic, but the time has come for us to be more honest. Losing breeder clients that do not follow best practice is no bad thing. By all means try to change them, but if it doesn't work say goodbye.

We need to focus on pre-purchase advice in any way we can. Client evenings for prospective puppy and kitten owners. Talk about the popular breeds. The brachy issues particularly are soul-destroying and the rocketing popularity needs tackling immediately. Talk about extremes of conformation and the impact it has on the lives of the animals.

We need to be leaders when it comes to not promoting deformed animals on practice social media and marketing materials. How many practice Facebook pages have the cute and cuddly Frenchies that came in plastered on the page rather than pointing out the disease and suffering? How many of us have colleagues who are vets and nurses that are buying or even breeding some of these worst-affected breeds? We have to be accountable as much as the next person.

As vets we are supposed to report corrective surgery and C-sections to the KC for registered animals. We all know there are 'brachy-friendly' clinics doing the vast majority of this stuff. They need to be scrutinised by the KC and the RCVS alike because if those practices are not reporting enormous numbers of operations then something needs to be done.

YOU!

There are a multitude of things that could make a huge difference to the health of our cats and dogs, but the parties involved are taking way too long to act. You, however, you have the power to make a change right now. By making the right choice about which animal you get you can improve animal welfare overnight. Consumers wield the ultimate power. If the demand for ill animals plummets only good can come of it in the long term.

Chapter 15

Staying Friends

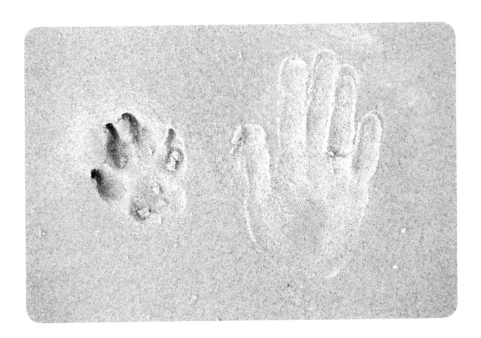

Acording to the Collins online dictionary, a friend is someone regarded with liking, affection and loyalty. I'd like to think this is how the majority of us see our pets. For many they are also part of the family and, whatever your feelings about seeing them like children, they are indeed like children in certain respects. They rely on us for everything after all. We teach them to trust us and that we will provide for them, protect them and not hurt them.

Our lives with animals, and children, should be based on mutual trust and respect. They should be friendships or relationships in which no one comes to any harm wherever possible. A friendship in which all parties gain happiness.

As I said all the way back at the beginning, this wonderful friendship of ours with dogs and cats has been formed over tens of thousands of years, but I fear that it has become an abusive relationship and all of the abuse is being meted out by us. I don't mean physical abuse here in the sense that everyone would judge as wrong.

I'm talking about abuse that, for many like me, is just as stark as physical abuse and we need to start seeing it as that. Some breeds of dog and cat are considered ancient, but look back at what we have done in those last few universal seconds of our beautiful friendship.

Because of our desire to manufacture animals at our whim, based on arbitrary, made up descriptions, we have fundamentally let these friends down. True friends care deeply about each other. They want the longest, healthiest life for each other. This way they get to spend more time together.

The concept of breed standards based on appearance not health is a major cause of suffering that is absolutely undeniable. In fact, in many developed countries I would go as far as to say that where pedigree numbers of dogs outstrip mongrels it is the biggest cause of suffering.

Every single phrase in a standard that calls for an abnormality or a defect should be seen for what it is – morally indefensible. I used this term in the last chapter, but I use it again here because we need to reflect on it. We have to start prioritising health and temperament way above what animals look like. We can have big dogs and small dogs and slightly different coats, but the time has come to stop dictating what they need to look like and start breeding the healthiest ones we've got left with each other. As far as cats go, I reiterate what I said in Chapter 13 – the selecting a kitten chapter – we do not need pedigree cats. In fact we need to stop the lunacy there right now. Cats are a wonderfully adapted and robust species. We can't top that and we should stop trying. Anyone breeding an extreme Persian or a Munchkin cat, or any number of extreme dog breeds we've mentioned, should be prosecuted for causing unnecessary suffering. If we set out to deliberately produce human offspring with this level of deformity and inherited disease there would simply be no question about it. It is *indefensible.*

Animals have no idea about social stigma, they don't understand why they have been dealt a certain body shape or a genetic make-up so they just get on with life, often with no complaints. The fact that animals can *cope* with an inadequate, frustrated, painful life does not make it a life worth living and certainly not one to strive for. We have a duty to ensure that every animal in our care has the chance to have the healthiest life we can give them. Thousands of vets all over the world are devastated by the day-to-day job of picking up the pieces of these sad lives. Lives that have been categorically changed for the worse because of human stupidity and vanity.

The showing of dogs, and especially, of highly territorial, easily stressed animals such as cats, needs to be stopped. Showing animals to judge them on how they look achieves nothing for the animal. Dogs may look excited after they've been in the ring, but simply praising a dog makes it act this way, it doesn't mean it enjoyed the experience. We have to start thinking about our animals selflessly. Does a rosette or a title really mean anything to your cat or dog? Would they have rather been tearing about in the woods or curled up by the fire? Do we honestly think that having your body prodded and poked and your genitals mauled by a stranger on a weekly basis is a pleasant or acceptable thing to put a beloved friend through? Certainly sounds abusive to me …

This friendship of ours needs rebooting like a computer program with a glitch. Our dogs and cats deserve more from us, don't they? We've changed so much in the blink of an eye, maybe through ignorance at the start, but we can't claim this as an excuse anymore. We need to act right now and in no uncertain terms to make sure the next blink of an eye, the next few decades, sees rapid and unquestionable movement away from disease and deformity towards health and happiness and lives truly worth living.

It all comes back to you. You are the future of dog and cat ownership. You can make that change happen right now by making the right choices about the life you want your pet to have. Ask yourself this. Will *you* be a good friend?

Acknowledgments

For many years I have continued this campaign and have received some fairly horrible abuse over the years from those who disagree with me. That said, alongside that abuse, I have had the enormous support and help of many friends, family and colleagues. For that I am deeply grateful. Those of you who have counselled me through the extreme lows, sat with me in the pub while I've cried, told me not to stop, but to see it through, sent me notes signed from the world's pugs; you are my great friends. Thank you.

This book *may* have been possible without the following people but it would not have been as accurate or as full of such wonderful images to get my point across! So I extend huge thanks for their time and effort to Jon Wray, David Gould, Nick Morton, Paul Joynson-Hicks, Dr Fraser Hale, Jane Ladlow, Nai-Chieh Liu, RSPCA, Andy Moores, Anna Porter, Jens Ruhnau, Kate Price, International Cat Care, IFAW, Cassie Smith, Carol Fowler, Charlotte Mackaness, Margaret Carter, the Dog Breeding Reform Group, Clare Rusbridge, Penny Knowler, Louise Engberg of www.klassiskperserkat.dk, Tanya Banks, Alex Gough, Dan O'Neill, Emma Bennett, Sheila Nolan, and CRUFFA.

Massive thanks also to Sara Davies, Karen Wild and Vicky Halls for their behavioural expertise and time.

Index

Pages numbers in *italics* refer to a figure.

hypertrophic cardiomyopathy (HCM)
96
hypoglycaemia (low blood sugar) 84

IFAW *see* International Fund for Animal
Welfare
inbreeding 7–8, 110–11
inherited problems 93–4, 104–5, 147
heart disease 94–6
intestinal problems 104
joint disease/skeletal problems 99–104
kidney/bladder problems 97–8
skin disease 96–7
injury
eyes 23, 24
protection from 120–1, 136–7
insurance companies 160
intensive farming 9
International Cat Care 35, 79, 145
International Fund for Animal Welfare
(IFAW) 112
intestinal problems 26, 104
Irish water spaniel 76
Irish wolfhound 85, 87, 124

Jack Russell 29, 33, 58, 85, 110
Japanese chin 12, 124
joint problems 87, 90, 99–104, 114

Kennel Club 10, 29–30, 31, 40, 44, 63, 75,
82, 88, 92, 93, 95, 108, 147–8, 150,
153–5, 159–60
kidney problems 97–9
King Charles spaniel 12, 124
kittens, choosing 133–4
breed health 139–40
breed/moggie characteristics 140–1
diet and fresh water 135–6
finding 133, 142–3
kept with/without other animals
137–8
normal behaviour 138
protection from pain, injury, disease
136–7
signs of health 144–5
socialisation and habituation 143–4
suitable environment 136
welfare needs 134–8
what to ask 144–5
knee problems 84
Komondor 75, 76

Labradoodle 114
Labrador (retriever) 47, 53, 59, 87, 97, 99,
110, 126, 147, 148
'Labrador tail' 59
LaFrance, Kay 34
laws/legislation 57, 59, 60, 125, 134,
157–9
legs 3
breed standards 22
luxated 31, 33, 82, 99
short 29, 30, 31, 34–5, *38*, 99
twisted/deformed 30–1, *32*, 35
Leonberger 85
Lhasa apso 47, 76, 97
life expectancy 85–6, 88, 153–4
line breeding 92
lips
covered by hair 77
drooping 40
liver shunts 84
long backs 29–30
Lowchen 76
luxating patellae (slipping knee caps) 31,
33, 82

Maine Coons 90, 96
Maltese terrier 76, 82
Manx cats 101–2, 140
mastiffs 40, 85, 90, 97, 110, 124
Michell, A.R. 85
miniature poodle 33
miniature schnauzers 97, 104
mitral valve disease (MVD) 95, 96, 152–5
moggies (cats) 2, 43, *70*, 86, 90, 94, 111,
115, 140–1
mongrels (dogs) 55, 73, 87, 94, 110–11,
112, 114, 115
Munchkin cats 34–5, 99, 140

Neapolitan mastiff 41, 87, 124
Newfoundlands 12, 85, 87, 90, 97, 124
Northern Ireland Welfare of Animals Act
(2011) 134
Norwegian forest cats 96

obesity 22, 30, 120, 122, 136, 156
obstructive airway disease 13, 156
OCD 87, 99
ocicats 97
O'Grady, Paul 81
Old English sheepdog (OESD) 63–4, 72, 76